WENDY Q. WANG

The Best Doctor
In You

The Body's Vital Energy Field, Pathways and
Acupuncture Points
Jingluo Therapy You Can Do Yourself
A Precise Handbook For Good Health And Longevity

E-West Publishing Company

The Best Doctor In You

Disclaimer

The Do-it-yourself Jingluo therapy described in this book is based on the theory and practice of Chinese Traditional Medicine. It is not intended to be a substitute for personal medical care and advice. You should always consult a healthcare professional about any health condition. Pregnant women should avoid it since it involves pressing, pounding, etc. That activity may complicate pregnancy. Also, if you are currently under any medication, please consult with your medical provider before engaging any actions. For underage children, parents have to be very gentle when giving massage to them. Pay attention to their reactions. Don't force the massage on them if they don't like it. Before starting any therapy program, also consult with your individual physician.

Published by:
E-West Publishing Company
Naperville, IL
www.e-westpublishing.com

ISBN 978-0-615-33629-9

Printed in China
First Paperback Edition

Dedication

**To my dear mother
who has given her whole life to us**

Acknowledgments

My family is my rock. My father, my two sisters, and my husband have always been there for me.

My older sister, Qingyuan, has suffered from rheumatoid arthritis for many years, but always keeps her spirits high and has a warm heart for living life. She taught herself computer graphic design and software applications and built a remarkable career. The pictures in this book are her work.

My younger sister, Qingtao is a talented architect. She has helped me in more ways than I can count. Some of the sketches in this book are her works.

My two sisters are my best friends. They support me in every way possible whenever I need a boost.

My dear father is the man I admire the most! His intelligence and diligence and his strong sense of responsibility to the family has set the highest of standards for my own life.

And of course, there is my dear husband Jeff, who is also my best friend. He has given me so much love and support all these years.

I am so grateful to have them all in my life!

I also want to thank my friends. They helped, encouraged and inspired me on my journey!

A special thank you goes to my editor, Linda Kleinschmidt, who did a fantastic job on this book and made it look better.

Contents

Preface

For many years, I wondered about one question: Why is life such a sad story for most of us? When we are young and full of energy, we lack wisdom and resources. We spend the prime of our youth working hard to build our lives. Years later, the lives around us start to be the way we want them to be. However, we begin to have less energy to enjoy what we have achieved fully. This is what time does to us. It gives us wisdom and resources, but then ages us and draws energy away from us, little by little and day by day.

Does life have to be this way? Why can't we prolong our optimal physical condition to the time when our wisdom climaxes and lives come together? Being smart and bright does not equal to wisdom. Wisdom does not happen without three elements. Those elements are - time, experience, and knowledge.

- Wisdom gives you intelligent ways of thinking about and looking at the world;
- Wisdom makes you understand all you did not understand before;
- Wisdom lets you value the real treasures you find in life and discard the meaningless parts of life even if they look attractive on the surface;
- Wisdom gives you peace; and
- Wisdom lets you enjoy life to the fullest.

Can we have the wisdom of our forties or fifties and also the energy level of our twenties? I have being looking for that answer, and now I believe the answer is YES. We can have both.

We all have been enjoying life with the help of modern technologies and the abundance of food that comes with many choices. We believe in the power of Western medicine for curing disease. However, we cannot help but notice that even with more and more resources spent on health care, people are not getting healthier. We've seen many cases where powerful drugs kill diseases and weaken a patient's body too much. The strong side effects of drugs make us wonder what the real sickness is.

About two yeas ago, I bought a book titled *The Handbook of How to Use Jingluos in the Human Body* by Dr. Xiao Yansheng. I had heard of Jingluos since I was little, but never had the curiosity to try to understand it. To me, and likely for most people, it was just a concept related to Chinese traditional medicine, which is always a back-up plan if we were sick. My knowledge to Chinese traditional medicine was also limited to doctors' making a diagnosis by feeling the pulse, and the smelly bitter herb medicine which had to be boiled very slowly to use. In the fast-paced modern society today, Chinese traditional medicine seemed to be out of date, and only had little value to add to our health and wellbeing.

Dr. Xiao's book gave me a whole new view of this ancient and amazingly profound theory about the human body. The more I studied it, the more curious and inspired I became. I started to research Jingluos and related areas and found I was entirely enjoying my new passion.

It all comes down to the understanding of our own body.

It all comes down to the circulation of energy in our body. The energy in our body has its particular routes to travel to supply the needs of every body part. Our human body is a brilliant system, and yet we misuse it even abused it too often. That is the reason why we have so many health problems and solved problem often bring out new ones. The cause for this vicious cycle is that the root of the problem is not handled properly. If we understand how our body works and keep the energy pathways open and efficient, our health will also improve significantly. The years we live with a good energy level will also increase considerably. Even 120 years of healthy life will no longer be impossible and unreachable. In our forties and fifties, we will still be just teenagers!

In this book, I talk about energy and Jingluos in a very straightforward way. The concepts are not mysterious once you look closely. I also introduce a number of acupuncture points and their helpful functions. In Chapter Four, I summarize over thirty Jingluo therapy methods to prevent and treat some of the most common diseases. These methods are practiced and taught by some of the most accomplished Chinese medicine doctors. This book is, therefore, titled, The Best Doctor In You. You and your Jingluos are the best doctors you can use.

Jingluo theory and Jinglou therapy for health care is an ancient and profound discovery about the human body. Such a remarkable finding should be recognized by all people in the world. Everybody should benefit from it. It will be a true blessing, if my work can accomplish just a little of that task.

Wendy Q. Wang
September 12, 2009

Chapter 1
Let's Explore Jingluo-What Is It?

1. Our Energy And The Jingluos

Life is all about energy. Without energy, there is no life. The world is run by energy, and so is our human body.

There are two types of crucial flows circulating inside our body. They are energy and blood. In Chinese medicine, the energy flow is called "Qi" (pronounced "chi"). We all know how important blood is, it is the fluid of life, but energy is the driving force. Each individual human body is an active energy field. That energy flows to reach every part of the body to support human life. The pathways that energy circulates through are called Jingluos. They are so vital that they decide how well we live, and in the end, they decide both life and death.

You see, when energy flows though Jingluos without obstacles, each part of the body gets just the right amount of energy to work well. The heart gets energy to pump enough blood into our vessels; the brain gets the right amount of energy to command muscles and organs to finish their jobs properly; and our bones are strong because of a sufficient energy supply. Our body is in a state of harmony. This harmony is the optimal health condition and we should do everything we can to keep the state that way for as long as we can.

When the pathways start to clog, the energy flow slows down. The energy cannot be transported to its destinations in time nor in a sufficient amount. Our body parts can't work properly. We don't have enough energy and motivation to be active. The whole body doesn't feel well and becomes very susceptible to disease. Without an adequate amount of energy and blood, our organs and body parts start to deteriorate. This is when our health starts to compromise and when we have to act to improve our physical conditions, it is not too late yet.

As more and more Jingluos are blocked, more and more body parts cannot obtain enough energy and blood. One under working or failed body part will affect others, create more blockages, and result in more under-working or failed body parts. Less and less energy is generated, and less and less fresh blood runs through the body. The vicious circle hence continues until there is no energy being transported at all. That is the end of life.

2. What Are The Jingluos, Acupuncture Points And Yin/Yang?

So, what are Jingluos and how do they work? How do we protect them from being blocked and keep them open and efficient to achieve good health and longevity?

As said before, Jingluos are the energy pathways inside our body and acupuncture points are the responsive or sensitive points on the Jingluos. Jingluos actually are Jings and Luos. Jings mean meridians or main pathways. They run longitudinally along the body. Each one belongs to one of the organs (only the twelve main meridians are associated with organs) and each one reflects a nature or aspect that is either Yin or Yang. Yin is moon and means darkness, coolness, moistness, and peacefulness. Yang is sun and means brightness, dryness, warmness, and liveliness. Yang is sky, and Yin is earth; Yang grows everything, Yin shapes everything. The balance of Yin and Yang is crucial. Too much or too little of either will cause disease. Luos mean network. They are the branches and sub-branches of the energy pathways. They spread all over the body, so energy can be transported everywhere.

Unlike blood vessels, Jingluos are invisible. There are no physical conduits or channels through which the flows run, but they do exist, just like the magnetic field of the earth which is invisible. The magnetic lines of force can not be seen by human eyes, but they stretch from the north to the south magnetic poles of the earth. Any pair of magnets will produce a magnet field with the magnetic lines of force curving from one to the other. If you cut through these lines with a conductor, electricity will be generated. This is how an electricity generator works. For more of information about this process, you have to study physics or electricity. Western medical people have tried to find Jingluos though autopsies, but this approach seems to be misleading. Since a dead body does not have any energy flow, how can you find Jingluos? just like an out-of-magnet field, you will not find the magnetic lines of force in it. However, when using a device to measure electrical resistance (R) and thermal sensitivities on a human body, the locations where Jingluos arc will have lower electrical resistance values, and the thermal contour lines coincide with the Jingluos on some parts of the body.

3. The History Of Jingluo Therapy

You cannot talk about Jingluo without mentioning the masterpiece written 2500 years ago in ancient China, called, *The Yellow Emperor's Classics of Internal Medicine*. This book discusses not only physiology, pathology, the diagnosis and treatment of disease, but also astronomy, geology, and philosophy. *The Yellow Emperor's Classics of Internal Medicine* states that everything that exists is related, and you can't make accurate conclusions by isolating one subject. At that time, people didn't have the tools we have today, such as fancy devices and instruments to detect diseases and other phenomenon in the universe. People then tried to understand the nature and the body by observing, listening, and feeling. They considered the human body as part of nature, part of the universe, and all should obey the laws and orders of that universe. In this book, Jingluos are given such crucial roles that they become the reasons why humans live, die, become sick, and thankfully also get well.

Therefore, taking care of the Jingluos especially before disease strikes and keeping them fluent all the time is the key to staying healthy. As one of the earliest people to practice Jingluo therapy, the Yellow Emperor lived to the age of over 100! Most of his descendants also enjoyed healthy long lives.

The theory of Jingluo did not stop there. With thousands of years of practice, perfection, and many remarkable medical personnel adding their contributions along the way, Jingluo theory and Jingluo therapy became sophisticated and extensive. Today, they are gaining more and more attention and respect around the world.

There are many methods for Jingluo therapy. The most known and easiest method is massage. It can be done by others, or alone. We will introduce some simple methods for self- massage in this book. By understanding our body more fully and regularly treating ourselves with massage, we can keep our Jingluos in optimal condition. We can be our own best doctors .

4. The Distribution Of The Jingluos

Main Meridians

There are twelve main meridians (Jings). Each one belongs to one of the organs, namely: the heart, pericardium (a double-walled sac that contains the heart and the roots of the great vessels), lungs, stomach, spleen, kidneys, liver, large intestine, small intestine, bladder, gall bladder, and SanJiao. In Chinese medicine, Sanjiao is the container for all the organs. The names of these meridians are very significant. Each contains four pieces of information: where, the nature (Yin or Yang), how much Yin or Yang, and which organ each belongs to. The twelve main meridians exist in pairs, symmetric about the centerline of the body. We only study one of them for each pair, because the other one is the same. Here are the names of the twelve main meridians:

1. Tai Yin lung meridian of the hands
2. Yang ming large intestine meridian of the hands
3. Yang ming stomach meridian of the feet
4. Tai Yin spleen meridian of the feet
5. Shao Yin heart meridian of the hands
6. Tai Yang small intestine meridian of the hands
7. Tai Yang bladder meridian of the feet

8. Shao Yin kidney meridian of the feet
9. Jue Yin pericardium meridian of the hands
10. Shao Yang Sanjiao meridian of the hands
11. Shao Yang gallbladder meridian of the feet
12. Jue Yin liver meridian of the feet

Note: Hands and Feet indicate the locations of the meridians, hand refers to the upper body. The hand meridian runs into the arm and hand. Foot refers to the lower body and runs from the upper body into the leg and foot. The amount of Yin/Yang ranges from large to small: Tai Yin > Shao Yin > Jue Yin, Yang Ming > Tai Yang > Shao Yang. When a meridian is Tai Yin meridian, it has the strongest Yin energy in it, the Shao Yin meridian has medium amount of Yin energy in it and the Jue Yin meridian has minimum amount Yin energy. A Yang Ming meridian has the strongest Yang energy in it, the Tai Yang meridian has medium amount of Yang energy and the Shao Yang meridian has the smallest amount of Yang energy in it.

Energy circulates within the meridians by following the direction from 1 to 12 as numbered above. Each meridian has two hours of the most active time every day. We will present the detailed time for each specific meridian in Chapter 3 and Appendix I . Theoretically, it is best to work on the meridian during its most active time, but this is not practical for those meridians with an active time in the middle of the night. Therefore, for daily health care, you can do the work whenever you have the chance. For medical treatment purpose, follow your doctor's advice.

Eight Extraordinary Meridians

There are eight extraordinary meridians. Unlike the main

meridians, they do not belong to any specific organs, but rather play very important roles in connecting the 12 main meridians. They support the main meridians to help them realize their functionalities and regulate and balance energy and blood flows. If the main meridians are rivers, the extraordinary meridians are their reservoirs. They conserve when the main meridians are full of energy, they irrigate and nourish when there is a need. The basic information about the eight extraordinary meridians is shown in the table below.

Name	Location	Functionality
1. Conception Vessel	The front center line of the body	Regulates the energy within all the Yin meridians
2. Governor Vessel	The back center line of the body	Regulates the energy within all the Yang meridians
3. Chong Vessel	On both sides of the Upper body back to the spine, in front up to the mouth	Nourishes the energy and blood flow within the 12 meridians
4. Belt Vessel	Around the waist line	Confines the longitudinal meridians
5. Yin Link Vessel	From and along the inner sides of the lower legs going up to the throat	Regulates the energy within the six Yin meridians
6. Yang Link Vessel	From and along the outer sides of the lower leg going up to the neck and forehead	Regulates the energy within the six Yang meridians
7. Yin Heel Vessel	From the inner sides of the heels, along the inner sides of the legs, going up to the inner sides of the eyes	Regulate the movements of the body muscles and eyelids
8. Yang Heel Vessel	From the outer sides of the heels, along the outer sides of the legs, going up to the inner sides of the eyes	

The centerlines of the body are the locations of the governor vessel and conception vessel. Their roles in regulating the energy flows are so critical that, they are grouped with the other 12 main meridians and described as the 14 main meridians.

5. Why Jingluo Therapy?

For those of us who want to live our lives to the fullest, we are not satisfied with just not being sick. We want to be strong, energetic, and motivated. We want to think clearly and feel wonderful all the time.

You can't always rely on doctors to give you medicine pills. The best doctor is the one can cure you before you get sick. In fact, the human body has its own best defense system for health, and that is the Jingluo. Its capacity is tremendous. We need to take care of it and keep it intact. When the dark force is near or attacking, we will be able to defeat it and stay unharmed. We also want to boost its potential to achieve our optimal health. This is the best doctor in our body and this is why Jingluo therapy is so appealing.

The basic idea for Jingluo therapy is very straightforward. That is, it opens up the body's energy pathways and boosts its natural potential to let energy flow without any obstacles. There is always an adequate amount of fresh blood to be transported to every part of the body. Then all the components will put on their best performance. A long and youthful life is realized naturally.

Jingluo therapy can be complex and the technique can be demanding. However, the beauty is, it also can be simple and so easy to be performed by yourself. As long as you are persistent, you'll love the results. In this book, we will introduce the methods practiced and taught by some of the most accomplished Chinese Medicine doctors. Hopefully, this will give you the amazing tools to achieve good heath and longevity.

One of the most important aspects of Chinese Medicine is disease prevention. A good doctor should be able to detect the earliest signs of sickness and treat it before it gets serious. There is a fascinating more than 2500-year old story. In the Chunqiu dynasty, there was a legendary doctor named Bianque. One day, he went to the country of Cai. When he saw the king, he recognized that the king was sick, but the sickness was still minor because it was only on the skin. He told the king that he was sick and should be treated, otherwise the sickness would go deeper. The king ignored him since he had not felt anything yet. After that visit, Bianque saw the king a few more times, and each time he saw the sickness had gone deeper. Each time he asked to treat him. The king was annoyed and disregarded all his suggestions. Then one day, Bainque saw the king again. As soon as he laid eyes on the king, he turned and ran. The king was very puzzled, so he sent somebody to ask why. Bianque told the messenger that the king's disease had gone too deep into his body. It was in his bone marrow now, and there was no cure for it. He could not save the king anymore. Several days later, the king started to have severe pains and desperately looked for Bainque. Bianque had already run to another country. The king died soon afterwards.

This story tells us how important early detection and early treatment are. However, we can't go to the hospital every day. Even if we do, the machines are not necessarily able to find out what's going on in our bodies before the symptoms become more obvious. This is why we should be very responsible for ourselves by doing two things: 1. do anything to stay healthy so we don't get sick easily. 2. pay close attention to our own body, it will give us signals when the body is not well. With more understanding of our own bodies, we'll be more alert to these warning signals and address them as soon as possible.

6. Chinese Kung fu and Jingluo

Every body heard about Chinese Kung fu either from the action movies or some other ways. It is viewed by the world as the powerful and handsome martial arts. Kung fu, in general, means hard works or the capability achieved through hard works. It can specifically refer to the martial arts. It was originally developed and practiced for the purpose of strong body and good health.

One of the most important aspects of Chinese Kung fu is Qi Kung. Kung means Kung fu. Qi, we mentioned in the beginning of this chapter, means the energy in the body, therefore, Qi Kung is the ability to master and control the energy flow in the body or Jingluos. One first has to have the Jingluos that are completely open and free of flows in order to practice the Kung fu to control the energy. If you are capable of maneuvering your energy and driving it anywhere you like in the body, this means power and longevity for you. That, off course, is not an easy task.

In Chapter 3, we will visit the 14 main meridians one by one. For each meridian, we will discuss its functions, what possible diseases and symptoms that relate to it, and how to prevent and deal with them though Jingluo therapy.

Chapter 2
Acupuncture Points
And The Basic Therapy Techniques

1. What Are The Acupuncture Points?

The English translation of 'acupuncture points' is not very accurate. Acupuncture is one of the many healing methods used in traditional Chinese Medicine. It inserts fine needles into the sensitive points on the body to stimulate Jingluos to cure the disease. These sensitive points are called "Shuxue" or "Xuewei" in Chinese Medicine, meaning 'the transmitting points'. However, the name "acupuncture points" has been so widely used, there is no point to change it now for our discussion.

Acupuncture points are the responsive points or sensitive points on the meridians and other parts of the body. They are the special locations where energy is transmitted between the inner structures and the surface of the body. These points can reflect disease or unhealthy conditions by giving forth painful sensations when touched or pressed. These points are (but not limited to) where the therapists apply treatments. When the body is deficient of positive energy, negative or harmful energy will be able to invade the body through the acupuncture points, causing illness. Stimulating the related acupuncture points can boost and mobilize the positive energy, balance Yin/Yang energy and cure

11

the disease.

There are three types of acupuncture points:

1. 14-main-meridian points
2. Extraordinary points
3. 'Yes' points.

The 14-main-meridian points are the points on the 12 main meridians plus the points on the governor and conception vessels. Each point has a unique name and a fixed location. They are the main acupuncture points.

The extraordinary points are the points that have names and fixed locations. These locations are not on a particular meridian. 'Yes' points are also called pain points, but they don't have names or fixed locations. They are the sensitive points related to the diseases. The 'yes' name came from a story. When treating a patient, the doctor pressed a spot unintentionally, and the patient uttered 'oh yes'.

There are approximately 360 acupuncture points in total on the human body. With so many tiny points to remember, one can easily be intimidated. As a matter of fact, for self -healing and caring purposes, we don't have to memorize all these points. We only need to remember roughly 20 most used and effective points. If you need to use more points, just look for them using the acupuncture point map. In Chapter 3, we will show all the acupuncture points on each meridian with accompanying pictures.

Each acupuncture point has a unique and meaningful name, which gives some key information about this particular point, such as main function, usage, location, or other. In English, the English spelling of the Chinese names are directly used. For people who don't understand Chinese, it is hard to comprehend the significance of each name and, therefore hard to remember all the foreign sounding names. In this book, we include the international symbols for all the listed acupuncture points. They are all shown on the sketches for each meridian (Jing) in each section in Chapter 3. We also indicate both the Chinese name and its English symbol in the title of the illustration for each particular acupuncture point. This information should provide more help.

The format of the international symbols for acupuncture points is also fairly easy. Since the most of the acupuncture points belong to one specific meridian (Jing), it only makes sense that their symbols are associated with those meridians. You can take two abbreviation letters of that meridian's name and number all the points along the way, from the starting point to the end point. For example: the name of the Xue-hai point means 'the sea of blood' in Chinese and can be used for blood-related issues. Its English symbol is SP10, because it belongs to the spleen meridian and is the 10th point from the start.

2. How To Find An Acupuncture Point?

When considering an acupuncture point as a tiny point, it might be really difficult to find it. However, if you think of it as a small precise area, it becomes quite easy.

To locate a subject on a 2D plane, you need 2 coordinates. To locate an acupuncture point, we use a reference point and a distance. The reference point is a known location on the body, such as 'the tip of the nose', 'the highest point of the ankle bone' etc. The distance is measured by your own hand. The unit is 'Cun'(see Figure 2-1).

How do you know if you have found the right acupunc-

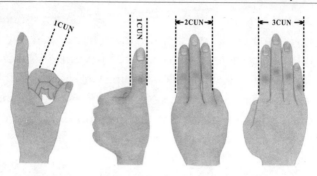

Figure 2-1 (Hand measurement: Cun)

ture point? When you press on it, if you feel kind of sore and sense a little pain (acute pain means you are not well somewhere), then you are on the right spot.

Every main meridian has a primary point. That is the point where the primary energy of this meridian originates. Stimulating this point is one of the most effective ways to boost the positive energy found in this meridian. We'll give the names and locations of these primary points in Chapter 3 as we go through each of the meridians one by one.

3. The Basic Therapy Techniques

1. <u>Pushing</u>: Using fingers (mostly thumb, index finger, and middle finger), whole hand or elbow, press on the targeted location and push parallel to the skin. This method helps circulate blood, relax the muscles and adjust energy flows in the Jingluos.

When operating, don't use too much force. The amount of force should depend on how your body feels. Feeling painfully comfortable is good. Push a little harder when exhaling and a little softer when inhaling. If you are young and strong, try using more force. For older people or weaker bodies, take it easy.

2. Rubbing: Using fingers, or palm, rub the area to warm. This activity can help accelerate the circulation of the blood, relax the skin and muscles, and get rid of coldness. This technique can be done on a relatively large area and for a relatively longer period of time.

3. Massage: Using fingers or the palm, press onto the aimed spot and move in a circular way. This procedure helps to circulate blood, unblock Jingluos, remove coldness, and relax the muscles. The force to be applied should always depend on how the patient feels and should not be too rough.

4. Tweaking: Using index finger and middle finger, or thumb and index finger, pinch and squeeze the skin. This action improves the circulation and relaxes the body. If you apply too much force, this tweaking will give you bruises. Be very careful.

5. Striking: Close both of the hands, beat the area with the outer edges of the closed palms. This action can relieve fatigue and clear Jingluos. The technique is mostly used on the head by other people. You can do this on the legs for yourself. Again, be careful with the force you apply.

6. Knocking (beating) meridians: Using your fist or a small massage hammer (usually made of wood or rubber), gently and with a steady rhythm, beat or tap along the meridians. The vibration produced by this action stimulates the entire beaten meridian to unblock the pathways and release energy flow. Be careful when using a small massage hammer. Do not use too much force. You could end up hurting yourself if you hammer too hard. Always start with a very gentle motion and gradually add strength, if pre-

15

ferred.

These are some of the easiest and the most commonly used techniques without tools to use for Jingluo therapy. There are many more complicated methods you can use with or without tools. For example:

- Stepping: The therapist stands on the body of the patient to do the treatment.
- Moxibustion: Using smoking moxa to warm the acupuncture points. Moxa is a stick with a shape looks like a cigar. It is made of dried plant called wormwood or Asiaticwormwood. The smoke and the warmth produced by the moxa can stimulate and unblock the Jingluos and free the energy inside.
- Cupping: Place a vacuumed cup onto the skin to suck the coldness and dampness from the inside of the body.
- Acupuncture: Inserting thin needles into the acupuncture points.
- Scraping: Scratching the skin with massage oil and a piece of thin plank made of cattle horn.

A professional Chinese medicine therapist can treat you with different techniques based on your sickness and your health condition.

Chapter 3
The Fourteen Main Meridians

In this chapter, we discuss the 14 main meridians one by one. You will find the following information for each of the meridians:

- The travel route and its significance. Please note that the meridian travel route picture in each section only shows the portions that lie on the surface of the body. The portions inside of the body are described by words.

- The location and functions of the primary acupuncture point.

- The common health syndromes related to each particular meridian.

- Prevention and treatment methods. Some key acupuncture points and their main functions are presented. Please note that in practice, combinations of different points on the same or different meridians are often used together to achieve the best results. In Chapter 4, we will introduce some of the simple and effective therapy methods targeting common syndromes by using the techniques and acupuncture points we have learned already.

- The most active time of the day for each meridian.

- 'Cun' is used as the unit for the measurement of distance when locating an acupuncture point. Figure 2-1

17

demonstrates the definition of 'Cun' using your OWN hands.

- We include the international symbols for each acupuncture point for easier memory. See Chapter 2 to understand how these symbols are constructed.

1. The Tai Yin Lung Meridian Of The Hand – Better Breathing Better Health

Introduction

The Tai Yin lung meridian of the hand (the lung meridian) belongs to the lung. It contains strong Yin energy. The human lungs are complex organs. They are the essential part of the respiration system. Their primary responsibility is to exchange oxygen and carbon dioxide between the blood and the air we breathe. In Chinese Medicine, the lungs are in charge of all air-related issues. They will supply air if it is deficient; adjust the direction if the air going the wrong ways; get rid of unclean air, and nourish the body with clean air. The quality of the lungs can also affect our emotions. The lung meridian is mostly used to deal with respiration problems, such as coughs, asthma, etc.

As shown in Figure 3-1, the lung meridian starts from the mid-section of the abdomen. It goes down to the large intestine and turns back up, along the stomach, through the diaphragm, to arrive at the lungs. It then goes upward and comes out of the throat, streams down to the arm, along the inner side of the arm, ending at the tip of the thumb.

From this route, we can see, besides the lungs, that this meridian is also closely related to the stomach and the large intestine.

There are 11 acupuncture points on this meridian (total of 22 points on both sides). Its primary point is the Tai-yuan point. This point is on the inner side of the wrist, at the intersection of the wrist line and the extension line of the thumb where the pulse can be felt (Figure 3-2).

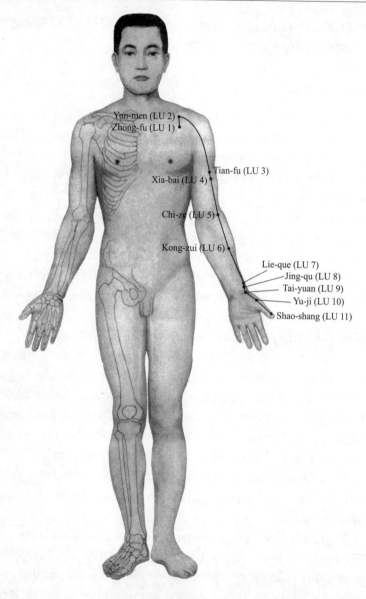

Yun-men (LU 2)
Zhong-fu (LU 1)
Tian-fu (LU 3)
Xia-bai (LU 4)
Chi-ze (LU 5)
Kong-zui (LU 6)
Lie-que (LU 7)
Jing-qu (LU 8)
Tai-yuan (LU 9)
Yu-ji (LU 10)
Shao-shang (LU 11)

Figure 3-1 (the lung meridian)

Common Syndromes Related To The Lung Meridian

Chronic tracheitis, bronchitis, asthma, chest pain, cough; uneasiness, frequent urine in small amount, stuffed nose, running nose, cold, abnormal skin blood circulation, dull skin color, arm and shoulder pain, muscle and joint pain along the meridian routes.

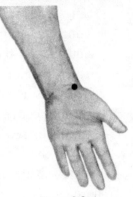

Figure 3-2
(the Tai-yuan point - LU 9)

Prevention And Treatment

- Massaging along the lung meridians will unclog the meridians. It will free the energy and let it reach everywhere in need. The lungs will function better, and lung diseases will be prevented.
- Tai-yuan point (Figure 3-2) deals with lung-related problems, especially cough. This is a key point for supporting breaths. If you always feel a shortness of breath or have weak breath, massage the Tai-yuan points more often. It will help you breathe more normally.
- Massage and press the Chi-ze and Kong-zui points:
Location: For Chi-ze point, bend your elbow. You'll find a tendon on the inner side of the arm. The recess inside of the elbow and on the thumb side of this tendon is the

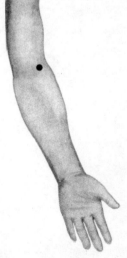

Figure 3-3
(the Chi-ze point - LU 5)

Chi-ze point (Figure 3-3).

- Kong-zui point is on the extension line of the index finger. 7 Cuns above the wrist line (Figure 3-4). Massaging these two points can heal cough, breath difficulty, chest pain, sore throat. These two points can be pressed harder to achieve better result.

The most active time for the lung meridian is 3 am to 5 am in the morning.

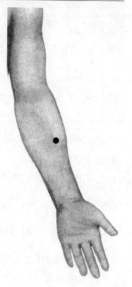

Figure 3-4
(the Kong-zui point - LU 6)

2. The Yang Ming Large Intestine Meridian Of The Hand – Keep The Body Free Of Waste And With Strong Immunity

Introduction

The Yang ming large intestine meridian of the hand (the large intestine meridian) belongs to the large intestine. It has very strong Yang energy. The large intestine is the final part of the digestive system. Its function is to absorb water from the remaining indigestible food matter and then pass useless waste material from the body. If the large intestine works appropriately, our body will not be filled with trash that will spoil our health. The large intestine meridian supplies the energy to let the large intestine carry out its task correctly.

The large intestine meridian starts from the tip of the index finger on the thumb side and on the back of the hand. It goes up, along the thumb side of the index finger, enters the back of the palm and then it goes into the forearm, elbow, upper arm, shoulder, and collarbone. It turns down, passes the lung to arrive at the large intestine. It has a small branch that comes out of the collarbone, goes up to the neck and chin, and then ends at the nose wing (Figure 3-5).

There are 20 acupuncture points on the large intestine meridian (a total of 40 points on both sides). The primary point is the He-gu point. It is between the thumb and the index finger on the back of the hand. When you close these two fingers, the highest point is the He-gu point (Figure 3-6).

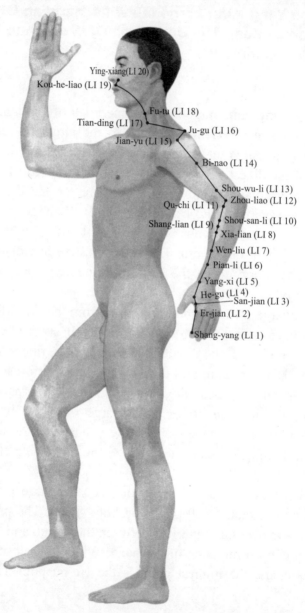

Ying-xiang(LI 20)
Kou-he-liao (LI 19)
Fu-tu (LI 18)
Tian-ding (LI 17)
Ju-gu (LI 16)
Jian-yu (LI 15)
Bi-nao (LI 14)
Shou-wu-li (LI 13)
Zhou-liao (LI 12)
Qu-chi (LI 11)
Shou-san-li (LI 10)
Shang-lian (LI 9)
Xia-lian (LI 8)
Wen-liu (LI 7)
Pian-li (LI 6)
Yang-xi (LI 5)
He-gu (LI 4)
San-jian (LI 3)
Er-jian (LI 2)
Shang-yang (LI 1)

Figure 3-5 (the large intestine meridian)

Common Syndromes Related To The Large Intestine Meridian

Common cold, bronchitis, fever, headache, cough, toothache, rhinitis, stuffed nose, sore throat, tinnitus, skin problems, muscle and joint pain occurs along these meridian routes.

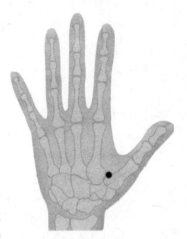

Figure 3-6 (the He-gu point - LI 4)

Prevention And Treatment

- The large intestine meridians are full of Yang energy. Regularly knocking along the routes can help detoxify blood, prevent acnes from growing, and strengthen immunity.

- Regularly massaging the He-gu points (Figure 3-6) can effectively prevent and cure the common cold, and increase immunity. The He-gu point is also an excellent painkiller and very effective for toothache, headache, and sore throat. Pressing He-gu points can relieve constipation as well.

- When bending the elbow, the end point of the elbow line on the thumb side is the Qu-chi point (Figure 3-7). It is great for relaxing a sore arm, relieving carpal tunnel syndromes, calming anxious and uneasy feelings. It can lower blood pressure and improve blood circulation.

- The Ying-xiang points: These are on the outer side and bottom of the nose wings (Figure 3-8). Useful for

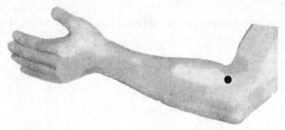

Figure 3-7 (the Qu-chi point - LI 11)

stuffed nose, chronic rhinitis, and allergic rhinitis. If you warm your fingers by rubbing them before you massage these points, you'll have better results.

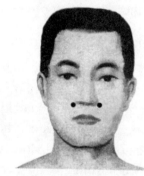

Figure 3-8 (the Ying-xiang points - LI 20)

The most active time for the large intestine meridian is 5 am to 7 am in the morning. Therefore, it is only natural for people to go to the bathroom in the morning during these hours.

3. The Yang Ming Stomach Meridian Of The Foot – The Most Vital Elements Built After Birth

Introduction

The Yang ming stomach meridian of the foot (the stomach meridian) belongs to the stomach. It has the strongest Yang energy and is one of the most important meridians in the body.

We have been talking about energy every step of the way so far, but what is the source of that energy? The answer is food. The food we eat has to be processed and converted into energy and then transferred among the Jingluos. The importance of what we eat and how we eat will be discussed in Chapter 5.

The stomach meridian belongs to the stomach and connects with the spleen. The stomach and spleen in Chinese Medicine together form the most important part of the digestive and absorption system. They work together to process the food we eat and convert it into energy, blood and nutrition that can be absorbed by the body.

It is from here, the stomach meridian, that the newly generated energy begins the journey of life. It travels around the body to supply every part of the Jinlous. This is how important the stomach meridian is. Without its good performance, everything else in the body is compromised.

From Figure 3-9, we can tell that the stomach meridian is a long stretch. It has two main lines and four branches. It has the most branches of all the meridians. It reaches the entire length of the body. The stomach meridian starts from the eye, circles around the face, and enters the mouth. It comes out of

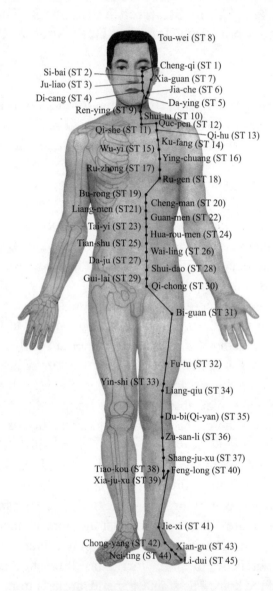

Figure 3-9 (the stomach meridian)

the lips, moves along the neck, goes down and through the diaphragm, arrives at the stomach and connects to the spleen. It then continues down, passes the belly button, streams into the leg, crosses the knee, and ends at the tip of the middle finger of the foot.

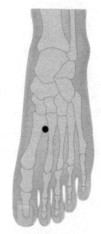

There are 45 acupuncture points on this meridian (a total of 90 points on both sides). The primary point is the Chong-yang point. It is the little dent right below the highest point on the back of the foot, between the toe and the second finger (Figure 3-10).

Figure 3-10
(the Chong-yang point - ST 42)

Common Syndromes Related To The Stomach Meridian

Stomachache, frequent yawning, fast heartbeat, agitation and craziness, stomach bloating, high fever, headache, neck pain, knee pain, easily hungry, easily scared by loud voices, nose bleeds, muscle and joint pains along the meridian route.

Prevention And Treatment

- Knocking on the entire or a portion of the stomach meridians for 10 to 20 minutes daily will keep the meridians uncongested. The energy can then flow efficiently inside. The stomach and other related organs will always be in good shapes and, therefore have strong immunity.

- Another great way to stimulate the stomach meridians is to push the entire abdomen. Starting from underneath the chest to the lower abdomen, use both hands to press on the body and slide down. There are many meridians going through this area. You will receive more benefit by massaging multiple meridians.
- The number one wellbeing acupuncture point: is Zu-san-li: it is on the outer front side of the lower leg, measuring 3 Cuns down from the bottom of the patella (knee cap) and right behind the tibia on the outer side (Figure 3-11).

Every Chinese Medicine doctor will tell you how important this point is. It has many responsibilities and can be extremely beneficial to your health if massaged regularly. First, it helps the peristaltic movement of the stomach and enhances the digestive function. Second, it regulates the heart rate and increases blood cells. Third, it helps the adrenal glands to work properly. This point is a wellbeing point, so every day 5 to 10 minutes of massage will keep you strong and slow aging. It is the No. 1 choice for treating all stomach problems. It also lowers the blood sugar level. It is better to use

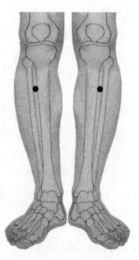

Figure 3-11
(the Zu-san-li points - ST 36)

some force when massaging the Zu-san-li point. The rule of thumb is to press on the point until you have a swelling sore kind of feeling.

- The Tian-shu points are on the same level as the belly button and 2 Cuns from it vertically. One is on each side. They can effectively relieve both diarrhea and constipation (Figure 3-12).

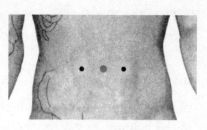

Figure 3-12
(the Tian-shu points - ST 25)

- The Si-bai points are below the eyes, on the line with the center vertical line of the eyes. The little dents on the cheekbones are these points. One on each side. They are very good for eyesight protection. They also improve blood circulation on the face. Regular massage of these points lets your face glow (Figure 3-13).

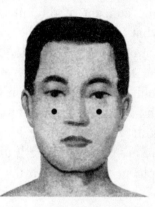

Figure 3-13
(the Si-bai points - ST 2)

The most active time for the stomach meridian is 7 am to 9 am in the morning.

31

4. The Tai Yin Spleen Meridian Of The Foot – The Body's Energy Generator

Introduction

The Tai Yin spleen meridian of the foot (the spleen meridian) belongs to the spleen. It is the strongest Yin energy meridian. The spleen is responsible for the destruction of redundant red blood cells, and holds a reservoir of blood. The concept of the spleen in Chinese Medicine is somewhat different from the spleen in Western medicine. It does not only reserve the blood but also turns the nutrients from the food into energy that will support our lives. It plays such an essential role in Chinese medicine that the spleen and the stomach are described as the most vital elements built after birth. The kidneys are the most vital elements we are born with, we'll discuss them in a later section. The spleen, together with the stomach, controls the generation of the energy and the blood and normalizes the digestive system. It has very powerful functions and, therefore, needs special care to maintain its high-quality working condition.

Figure 3-14 shows the route of the spleen meridian. The energy flow comes out of the stomach meridian and continues its journey here. It starts from the tip of the toe, goes up to reach the knee, along the inner side of the leg, climbs into the abdomen to then arrive at the spleen. It connects to the stomach, then keeps rising to the chest and the throat, ending at the tongue.

There are 21 acupuncture points on the spleen meridian (a total of 42 points on both sides). The primary point is

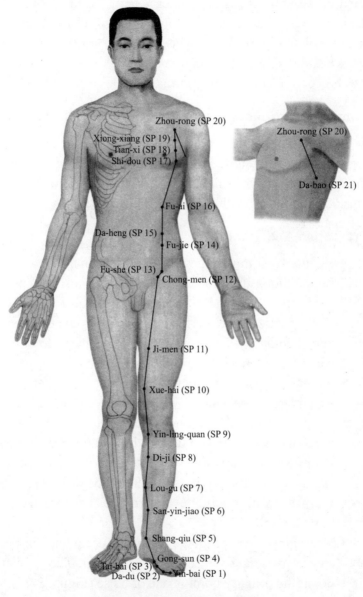

Zhou-rong (SP 20)
Xiong-xiang (SP 19)
Tian-xi (SP 18)
Shi-dou (SP 17)
Fu-ai (SP 16)
Da-heng (SP 15)
Fu-jie (SP 14)
Fu-she (SP 13)
Chong-men (SP 12)
Ji-men (SP 11)
Xue-hai (SP 10)
Yin-ling-quan (SP 9)
Di-ji (SP 8)
Lou-gu (SP 7)
San-yin-jiao (SP 6)
Shang-qiu (SP 5)
Gong-sun (SP 4)
Tai-bai (SP 3)
Da-du (SP 2)
Yin-bai (SP 1)

Zhou-rong (SP 20)
Da-bao (SP 21)

Figure 3-14 (the spleen meridian)

33

the Tai-bai point. It is at the inner side of the foot. The depression behind and below the highest point of the toe joint is this point (Figure 3-15). This is a very important point for a healthy spleen. It strengthens a weak spleen, regularizes bowel movements, and normalizes blood sugar levels.

Common Syndromes Related To The Spleen Meridian

Indigestion, diarrhea, constipation, stomach ache, bloating, fatigue, overweight, lose of appetite, stiff tongue, painful menstruation, irregular menstruation, pelvic problems, muscle and joint pain along the meridian routes.

Prevention And Treatment

- Regularly stimulating the spleen meridians by massaging along their routes will boost the positive energy level. It enhances the blood generation process and optimizes the performance of the spleen. It is very good for women's wellness and helps to solve weight problems (overweight and underweight).
- Eating too much especial fatty foods, will overwork the spleen. The spleen will become exhausted and worn-out and will no longer be able to keep up with the assignments. If you drool with a bad smell during sleep, you probably have eaten too much dinner. Massaging your Tai-bai points (Figure 3-15) will help.
- Keep a positive attitude toward life, because worry hurts the spleen.
- Massaging some of the key acupuncture points on the spleen meridians will be very beneficial. The Tai-bai point, the primary point is one of these (Figure 3-15).
- The Gong-sun point: is at inner side of the foot below

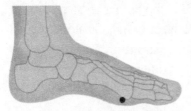   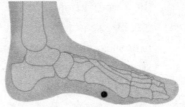

Figure 3-15 (the Tai-bai point - SP 3)   Figure 3-16 (the Gong-sun point - SP 4)

the foot bones, 1 Cun from the highest point of the toe joint, toward the ankle (figure 3-16). It is one of the important points for treating female diseases, such as painful menstruation, irregular menstruation, infertility. It also treats stomach pain, bloating, high blood pressure, numb hands, and back pain.

- The San-yin-jiao point: is on the inner side of the lower leg and behind the tibia, 3 Cuns above the tip of the ankle bone (Figure 3-17). This point is the intersection of the three Yin meridians (spleen, kidney and liver). It is very effective in treating female diseases. It regulates the blood by either stopping bleeding or unblocking blood circulation. It helps relieve painful menstruation and menopause syndromes. It deals with weight problems (overweight or underweight), and cold hands and feet.

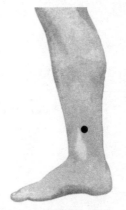

Figure 3-17
(the San-yin-jiao point - SP 6)

- The Xue-hai point: is on the front upper leg, 2 Cuns from the upper edge of the patella, on the inner side of the femur bone (Figure 3-18). The name of this point means 'sea of blood'. It treats all kinds of blood related illnesses, such as painful menstruation, irregular menstruation, bleeding, blood deficiency, etc.

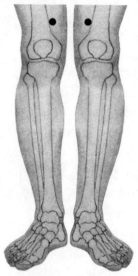

Figure 3-18
(the Xue-hai points - SP 10)

The most active time for the spleen meridian is 9 am to 11 am in the morning.

5. The Shao Yin Heart Meridian Of The Hand – The Controller Of The Mind

Introduction

The Shao Yin heart meridian of the hand (the heart meridian) belongs to the heart. It has medium amount of Yin energy. The heart controls the mind. You probably say, however, "Wait a minute! The brain controls the mind!" However, the heart controls blood flow, if the heart can't supply enough blood for the brain, your mind is not going to work! That's how significant the heart is and also the heart meridians.

As shown in Figure 3-19, the heart meridian starts at the heart. It goes down cross the diaphragm, connects to the small intestine; it then turns back up and reaches the lung and comes out of the armpit; then it steams down to the elbow and palm, ending at the little finger. It also has a small branch rising from the heart to the throat and eye.

There are 9 acupuncture points on the heart meridian (18 total on both sides). The primary point is the Shen-men point. There is a hard tendon along the little finger on the inner side of the wrist, the intersection of this tendon and the wrist line is the Shen-men point (Figure 3-20).

Common Syndromes Related To The Heart Meridian

Heart problems, such as coronary heart disease, angina, and irregular heartbeat; nervousness, trouble sleeping, neurasthenia, depression, forgetfulness, and muscle and rib pain along the meridian routes.

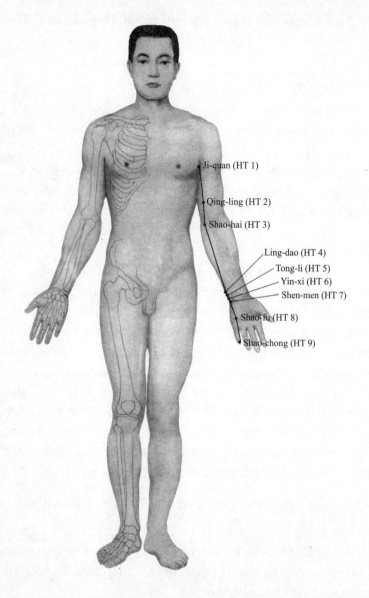

Figure 3-19 (the heart meridian)

Prevention And Treatment

- Regularly massaging along the heart meridians can prevent heart problems. It can minimize the chances of a heart attack, enhance mood, clarify the mind, and prevent and relieve depression. A healthy heart meridian also lets you rest well during the night.

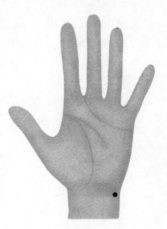

Figure 3-20
(the Shen-men point - HT 7)

- The Shen-men point is the primary point on the heart meridian (Figure 3-20). It prevents and treats heart disease, uneasiness, trouble sleeping, depression, forgetfulness. It calms the heart.

- The Ji-quan point is the highest point inside the armpit (Figure 3-21). This is a very good point for preventing heart disease. It improves the blood delivering process in the body. Plunking (press down and move the fingers horizontally) is a good way to stimulate this point.

- The Shao-hai point: at the bend in the elbow, extends in a line from the little finger. The intersection of this line

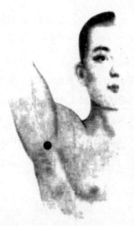

Figure 3-21
(the Ji-quan points - HT 1)

and the folding line inside the elbow is the Shao-hai point (Figure 3-22). It treats irritability and hotness in the night, trouble sleeping, heart pain, trembling or cramping hands, and tinnitus.

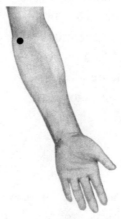

Figure 3-22
(the Shao-hai point - HT 3)

The most active time during the day for the heart meridians is 11 am to 1 pm. A short nap after lunch is a very healthy habit to practice. The heart will concentrate on cleaning up the waste and toxics in the meridians while you are resting. This is also the time when Yang energy and Yin energy switch their power and a short nap lets the heart rest a little without interrupting the transition of Yin/Yang energy.

6. The Tai Yang Small Intestine Meridian Of The Hand – The Manager Of The Body's Liquid

Introduction

The Tai yang small intestine meridian of the hand (the small intestine meridian) belongs to the small intestine. It has a good amount of yang energy. The small intestine is where the majority of digestion occurs. Most of the nutrients found within food are absorbed here. If the small intestine is not working properly, there will be problems. The small intestine meridian not only manages digestive functions, but also handles back and shoulder issues. If the heart is short of blood, the small intestine meridian will reflect it.

The small intestine meridian is in charge of body's liquids, such as menstruation, milk, gastric juice and other secretion from the glands. Therefore, you can always find solutions on the small intestine meridians for most of the liquid related problems.

From Figure 3-23, the small intestine meridian is on the outer side of the arm. It starts from the tip of the little finger, along the back of the hand, goes up to the forearm, elbow, and upper arm; then it goes around the shoulder, turns back down, crosses the heart, passes the stomach, and arrives at the small intestine. It has a branch coming out of the shoulder, rising up to the neck, ending at the ear.

There are 19 acupuncture points on the small intestine meridian, (38 total on both sides). The primary point is the Wan-gu point. It is on the back of the hand and on the little finger side. To find it, rise your fist upward, there is a hori-

41

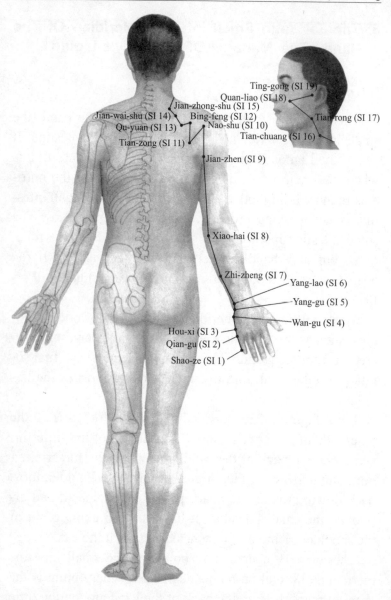

Figure 3-23 (the small Intestine meridian)

zontal line toward the bottom of the metacarpal bone of the little finger, the little dent behind this bone is this point (Figure 3-24).

Common Syndromes Related To The Small Intestine Meridian

Throat pain, eye pain, tinnitus and other hearing problems, headache; trouble sleeping, shoulder pain, epilepsy, muscle and joint pain along the meridian route.

Prevention And Treatment

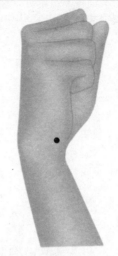

Figure 3-24
(the Wan-gu point - SI 4)

- Regularly massaging along the small intestine meridians can relax muscles and prevent and relieve cervical neck pains. It keeps the energy pathway open and ensures the small intestine and other related organs work right.
- The Wan-gu point (Figure 3-24) is the primary point. This point can regulate the functions of the small intestine, lower blood sugar level, treat headaches and tinnitus, and relive constipation.
- The Tian-zong point: it is a little above the center point of the shoulder blade and parallel to the fourth dorsal vertebra (Figure 3-25). This is a sensitive point. When pressing or massaging this point, you can feel a strong sore pain. For those who work at desks or use computers all the time, cervical neck pain is a very common syndrome. Symptoms like a stiff back and neck, pain and sore shoulders can cause severe problems if not

given enough attention. The Tian-zong points can help.

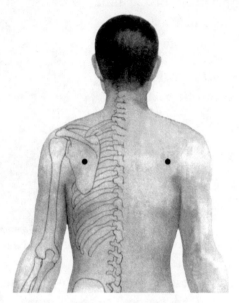

Figure 3-25 (the Tian-zong points - SI 11)

The most active time for the small intestine meridian during the day is 1 pm to 3pm in the afternoon.

7. The Tai Yang Bladder Meridian Of The Foot – The Body's Detoxification Route

Introduction

The Tai Yang bladder meridian of the foot (the bladder meridian) belongs to the bladder. It has a good amount of Yang energy. As we know, the body's three most important detoxification methods are urination, defecation, and perspiration. A human can live without defecation for 10 days. If a person does not urinate for three days, however, he or she will be in a very dangerous condition. The bladder meridian is in charge of both urinating and sweating. Therefore, the importance of this meridian is obvious. It also acts as a natural screen to protect our bodies from attack by harmful influences.

As shown in Figure 3-26, the majority of this meridian is on the back of the entire body. It has one main route and three branches. It starts at the inner corner of the eye, goes up to the top of the head, then along the back of the head, and reaches down to the back. It then connects to the kidney and arrives at the bladder. The longest branch comes from the back of the shoulder, travels down the leg and ends at the tip of the little toe.

There are 67 acupuncture pointes on each of these two meridians (134 points total). It is the meridian that has the most acupuncture points. It has a passage point to every major organ, such as Xin-shu (the heart passage point); Shen-shu (the kidney passage point); Fei-shu (the lung passage point), etc. The primary point is the Jing-gu point. It is on the little toe side of the foot and beneath the end of

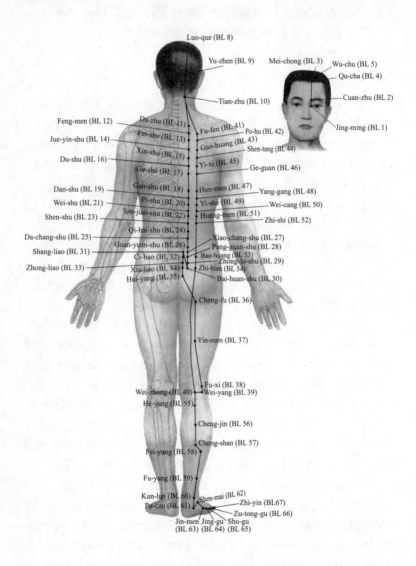

Figure 3-26 (the bladder meridian)

the fifth metatarsal bone (Figure 3-27).

Common Syndromes Related To The Small Intestine Meridian

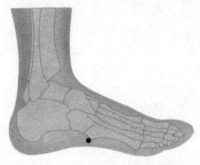

Respiratory system: Cold, fever, asthma, chronic or acute bronchitis, pneumonia.

Figure 3-27 (the Jing-gu point - BL 64)

Digestive system: Indigestion, dysentery, gastroptosis, gastroenteritis, hepatitides, and cholecystitis

Urinary system: Mephritis, impotence, painful menstruation, and irregular menstruation.

Other syndromes are trouble sleeping, back pain, arthritis, muscle pain along the meridian route.

Prevention And Treatment

- The bladder meridians are on the back side of the body. The portion on the lower body can be easily reached alone. You can use fists to pound on the hips and the back of the legs and all the way to the sides of the feet. Doing so makes sure energy and blood flow efficiently and keeps the detoxification path in a healthy state.

- The upper body portion of the bladder meridian is hard to reach alone. family members can help each other by doing back pinching. Let the person lie on his/her stomach. The other person will then use both hands to pinch both sides of the spine from the bottom of the spine all the way to the hairline (Figure

3-28). This equals one round, do 6 rounds every day. This is a really good way to take care of the bladder meridians. You are actually stimulating all the organ passage points we mentioned above. The functions of these organs will be normalized, and many of your discomforts and symptoms will disappear.

• Combing the hair frequently with a wooden or a cattle horn comb is an excellent way of massaging the bladder meridians. As you know, these meridians go through almost the entire head.

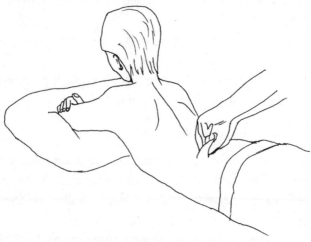

Figure 3-28 (back pinching)

The most active time for the bladder meridian during the day is 3 pm to 5 pm in the afternoon.

8. The Shao Yin Kidney Meridian Of The Foot – The Most Vital Elements That You Are Born With

Introduction

The Shao Yin kidney meridian of the foot (the kidney meridian) belongs to the kidney. It has a medium amount of Yin energy. The kidneys remove waste and extra water from the blood to form urine which is later drained out of the body. In the spleen meridian section, we mentioned that the stomach and the spleen are the most vital elements built after birth. The kidneys are the most vital elements that you are born with. Well functioning kidneys are the prerequisites for good health. If your parents gave you strong kidneys, you are very lucky. If you don't naturally have strong ones, you have to make an effort to strengthen them. In Chinese Medicine, the kidneys store the essence of life. They control growing, maturing, reproduction, and liquid circulation in the body.

The kidney meridian connects to more organs than any other meridians. Taking good care of the kidney meridians will keep the kidneys and the other organs in good working condition. The meridian starts from the bottom of the little toe, crosses the bottom of the foot, rises to the inner side of the ankle. Then, it moves along the leg, it climbs into the abdomen, passes the spine, arrives at the kidney, and connects to the bladder; It then comes to the front, continues to travel up to the lung, liver, diaphragm and the throat, and ends at the tongue. The branch at the lung connects to the heart and ends at the chest. (See Figure 3-29.)

There are 27 acupuncture points on the kidney meridian (a

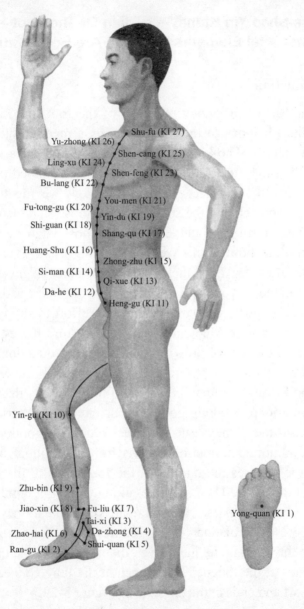

Figure 3-29 (the kidney meridian)

total of 54 points on both sides). The primary point is the Tai-xi point. It is placed in the middle of the recess behind the ankle bone (Figure 3-30).

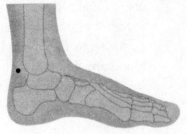

Figure 3-30 (the Tai-xi point - KI 3)

Common Syndromes Related To The Kidney Meridian

Chronic or acute prostatitis, impotence, premature ejaculation, spermatorrhea, testicle problems, painful menstruation, irregular menstruation, kidney problems, back pain, hungry but no desire to eat, weak back and weak lower body, and muscle and joint pain along the meridian routes.

Prevention And Treatment

- Massage the kidney meridians for 10 to 20 minutes daily, and at the same time, emphasize the key acupuncture points. This will open up the energy pathways and deliver plenty of energy to the kidneys and other organs. Your body will thank you by giving you long lasting vitality and youthfulness.
- The Tai-xi point (Fgure 3-30), is the primary point of the kidney meridian. It can boost the original energy of the kidney to carry the blood for circulation. This is a very important point for kidney care.
- The Yong-quan point is one of the most important wellbeing acupuncture points. It is on the bottom of the foot. To find it, cover all the toes. The recess on the upper 1/3 line is this point (Figure 3-31). The purpose for stimulating the Yong-quan point is to direct the

51

energy and blood to this point. With the aging process, the most noticeable phenomenon is that the legs are not as strong as they were before. Not enough energy and blood are able to travel all the way down the legs. The Yong-quan point can come to rescue. You can press on this point, massage it, or rub the entire foot bottom with your palm.

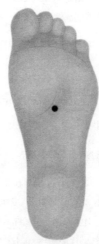

Figure 3-31
(the Yong-quan point - KI 1)

The most active time for the kidney meridian during the day is 5 pm to 7 pm.

9. The Jue Yin Pericardium Meridian Of The Hand – The Protector Of The Heart

Introduction

The Jue Yin pericardium meridian of the hand (the pericardium meridian) belongs to the pericardium. It has a minimum amount of Yin energy in it. The pericardium is a double-walled sac that contains the heart and the roots of that great vessel. It maintains the heart in its normal position and safeguards the heart from infection and reduces external friction. The pericardium acts as a protector of the heart. If it malfunctions, the heart is in danger. Having a healthy pericardium meridian reduces the chances of heart attack and other heart disease significantly. Caring for pericardium meridians is a life-saving task.

As shown in Figure 3-32, the pericardium meridian lies on the middle of the inner arm. It starts from the chest and proceeds to the pericardium; It then goes down through the diaphragm, connects to the Sanjiao (Sanjiao is the container of all the organs). The branch comes out of the chest to the underarm, along the inner arm, goes down to the hand, and ends at the tip of the middle finger.

There are 9 acupuncture points on the pericardium meridian (18 points total on both sides) and the primary point is the Da-ling point at the center of the wrist line (Figure 3-33).

Common Syndromes Related To The Pericardium Meridian

Nervousness, irregular heartbeat, angina, chest pain,

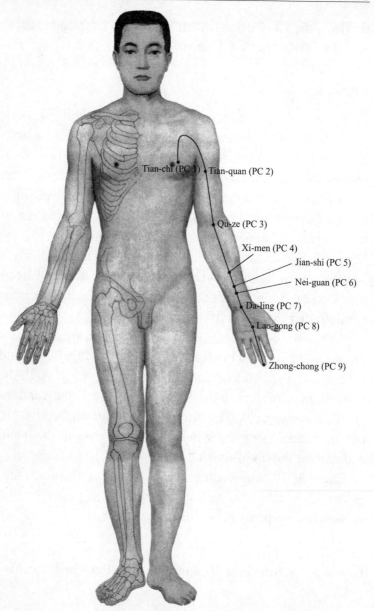

Figure 3-32 (the pericardium meridian)

trouble sleeping, depression, stomach ache, nausea, and muscle and joint pain along the meridian route.

Prevention And Treatment

- Massaging the pericardium meridians regularly keeps energy and blood circulating fluently and supplies the heart with a good amount of energy. It also helps to reduce fat build-up in the arteries and decreases the chances for heart

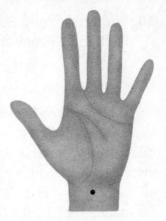

Figure 3-33
(the Da-ling point - PC 7)

disease. When massaging this meridian, do not use too much force, so as not to exceed your comfort level.

- The Da-ling point (Figure 3-33), the primary point, strengthens both the heart and the spleen. It can relieve sleeplessness as well.
- The Nei-guan point is 2 Cuns above the center of the wrist line. This is a very useful point. It calms the heart, stops pain, regulates blood pressure and heartbeat and also comforts the stomach. (Figure 3-34).

The most active time for the pericardium meridian during the day is 7 pm to 9 pm in the evening. You should not work on this meridian immediately after meals. Wait for at least half an hour.

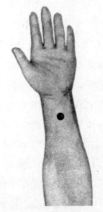

Figure 3-34
(the Nei-guan point - PC 6)

10. The Shao Yang Sanjiao Meridian Of The Hand – Relieving Pressure And Balancing Hormones

Introduction

The Shao Yang Sanjiao meridian of the hand (the Sanjiao meridian) belongs to Sanjiao. It has a small amount of Yang energy. Sometimes it is called the Triple Energizer meridian. Sanjiao, in Chinese Medicine, is the container of all the organs. It is divided into three parts, the upper Jiao, the middle Jiao and the lower Jiao. The upper Jiao contains the heart and lungs; the middle Jiao contains the spleen, stomach, liver, and gallbladder; the lower Jiao contains the kidneys, bladder, and large and small intestines. The Sanjiao is the general manager of all the organs, it coordinates the organs, so they work harmoniously together. The Sanjiao meridian links all these parts by transporting and distributing energy among them.

As shown in Figure 3-35, the Sanjiao meridian is on the back side of the arm. It starts from the tip of the ring finger, along the back of the hand, goes up to the elbow and shoulder. It then turns inside, connects the pericardium, crosses the diaphragm, and arrives at the Sanjiao. The branch comes out of the chest, moves along the side of the neck to the ear, around the back of the ear, then goes up, ending at the outer end of the eyebrow.

There are 23 acupuncture points on the Sanjiao meridian (46 in total on both sides). The primary point is the Yang-chi point. It is located on the back of the wrist; the little dent in the mid point of the wrist line is this point (Figure 3-36).

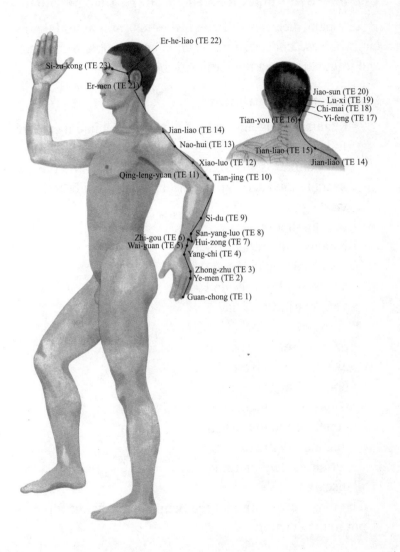

Figure 3-35 (the Sanjiao meridian)

Common Syndromes Related To The Sanjiao Meridian

Ear pain, hearing difficulty, tinnitus, migraine, hemifacial spasms, constipation, cold, elbow problems, muscle and joint pain along the meridian route.

Prevention And treatment

- Regularly massage and pat along the Sanjiao meridians to keep the energy flow going without obstacles. Since the Sanjiao is the general manager of all the organs, keeping this meridian in a healthy condition benefits all the organs. It normalizes the hormone level, balances the mood, relieves constipation, and keeps the skin around your eyes free of lines.

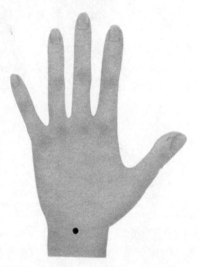

- Yang-chi point: This primary point (Figure 3-36), can activate the body's Yang energy. It is one of the main acupuncture points when treating diabetes and certain other chronic diseases.

Figure 3-36 (the Yang-chi point - TE 4)

The most active time for the Sanjiao meridian is 9 pm to 11 pm in the evening.

11. The Shao Yang Gallbladder Meridian Of The Foot – The Outstanding Health Manager

Introduction

The Shao Yang gallbladder meridian of the foot (the gallbladder meridian) belongs to the gallbladder. It has a small amount of Yang energy. The gallbladder is a small pear-shaped organ that acts as a storage vessel for bile. Bile is made by the liver and is the main substance responsible for breaking down fat in the digestive system. The gallbladder receives bile from the liver and stores it until a meal is eaten. The digestive system needs bile to be released into the intestine to dissolve fats and cholesterols. So the gallbladder is a very important element for digestion and detoxification. The gallbladder meridian carries a huge amount of toxic substances from the liver and is very easy to get congested. With a congested gallbladder, liver waste cannot be cleaned effectively either. Thus, the gallbladder meridian often needs to be unclogged. Knocking along the gallbladder meridians with your fists is a very good way to fulfill this need.

The gallbladder meridian runs on the side of the body and is the longest meridian. As shown in Figure 3-37, it starts from the inner corner of the eye, goes around the side of the head and ear, then drops down to the shoulder, ribs, and arrives at the gallbladder; it connects the liver and descends to the foot, ending at the tip of the ring toe.

There are 44 acupuncture points on the gallbladder meridian (totaling 88 points on both sides). The primary point is the Qiu-xu point. It is below the ankle and in the little dent

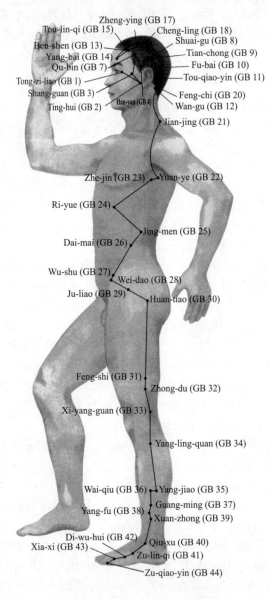

Figure 3-37 (the gallbladder meridian)

outside of the ring toe exten-
sor tendon (Figure 3-38).

Common Syndromes Related To The Gallbladder Meridian

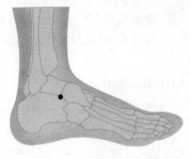

Figure 3-38 (the Qiu-xu point - GB 40)

Gallbladder problems, liver problems, ear and hearing
problems, migraines, bitterness
in the mouth, dull skin color, sighing all the time, breast
problems, muscle and joint pain along the meridian route.

Prevention And treatment

Using your fists, knock along the gallbladder meridians. It
is an effective and convenient way to increase the liver's
ability to secrete bile. It will reduce the possibilities of Jingluo congestion and avoid the toxins piling up in the liver and
meridians. Doing so helps to achieve psychological balance
as well. They are on the outer sides of the body and easy to
reach. Every night, before going to bed, knock on both sides
from the hips to the legs for about 10 minutes. It will benefit
not only the gallbladder, but also the liver significantly. It also
keeps you energetic during the day.

The most active time for the gallbladder meridian is 11
pm to1 am.

12. The Jue Yin Liver Meridian Of The Foot – Saving Life And Enhancing Mood

Introduction

The Jue Yin liver meridian of the foot (the liver meridian) belongs to the liver. It has a minimum amount of Yin energy. The liver is such a vital organ. It has a multitude of important and complex functions that support human life. From the section above, we learned that the liver produces bile for the digestive system to process the food we eat. The liver cleans the blood by removing waste products, worn-out cells, bacteria, and other poisonous substances in the bloodstream. It produces immune factors and resists infections and much more. The liver carries heavy loads every day not only from the things (food, liquor, drugs) we take, but also from the habits and emotions we experience, such as exhaustion and anger. If we keep ignoring our livers, some day, the liver will collapse causing devastating consequences. Fortunately, the liver meridian provides us with a powerful tool for liver care.

From Figure 3-39, we can see that the liver meridian is not very long and doesn't have many acupuncture points. It starts from the inner side of the big toe, goes up to the ankle, along the inner side of the leg, to get to the lower abdomen. It then keeps going upward, arriving at the liver and connecting to the gallbladder. Then it continues to cross the diaphragm, comes to the throat, passes the eye, and ends at the top of the head.

There are 14 acupuncture points on the liver meridian (totaling 28 points on both sides). The primary point is the

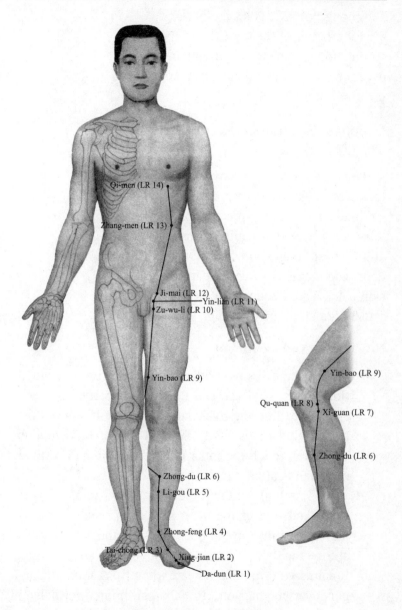

Figure 3-39 (the liver meridian)

Tai-chong point. It is on the back of the foot, between the big toe and the second toe, at the recess point between the highest point and the end of the toe (Figure 3-40).

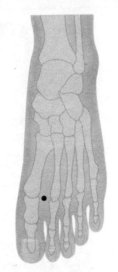

Figure 3-40
(the Tai-chong point - LR 3)

Common Syndromes Related To The Liver Meridian

Unable to stretch backwards due to lower back pain, liver problems, gallbladder problems, prostate problems, painful and irregular menstruation, chest congestion, bad temper, depression, enuresis, dry throat, dull skin color, also, frequently wake up at 1 to 3 o'clock in the morning.

Prevention And treatment

- Massage the liver meridians to let energy and blood flow freely, so liver can function properly. The easiest way to find the liver meridian is to stretch out the leg parallel to the body. You'll find a hard tendon when you touch the inner side of the thigh. The liver meridian is along this tendon.

- The Tai-chong point is the primary point (Figure 3-40) and one of the most important wellbeing acupuncture points on the body. It strengthens the liver's ability for detoxification, and lowers blood pressure. It calms your mind and heart when frustration and anger overwhelm you. It helps sleeping, normalizes menstruation, and improves sexuality. Regularly massaging this point will be very beneficial to your over-all wellbeing.

The most active time for the liver meridian is 1 am to 3 am in the morning.

13. The Conception Vessel – Nourishing Kidneys And Normalizing Sex Hormones

Introduction

The conception vessel is the centerline of the body on the front. It is one of the eight extraordinary meridians. Unlike the twelve main meridians, it does not belong to a particular organ. It is the controller of all the Yin meridians, regulating and normalizing Yin energy among them. It has a close relationship with the female reproductive system. In Chinese Medicine, kidney energy is the main driving force for the reproductive process; the actual place for birth is the uterus. The conception vessel is the connection between the organs and the uterus. The conception vessel is a very good resource for strengthening the kidneys, normalizing sex hormone levels, and enhancing sexuality.

As shown in Figure 3-41, the conception vessel starts from inside the lower abdomen (if female, it starts from the uterus). It comes out of the perineum, along the centerline of the upper body, rises up to the throat, goes around the mouth, and ends underneath the eyes.

There are total 24 acupuncture points along the conception vessel. The meridian is related to the nervous system, respiratory system, digestive system, urinary system, and reproductive system

Common Syndromes Related To The Conception Vessel

Painful menstruation and various other female-related problems, prostatitis, impotence, premature ejaculation, stomachache, indigestion, trouble sleeping, chest congestion, and

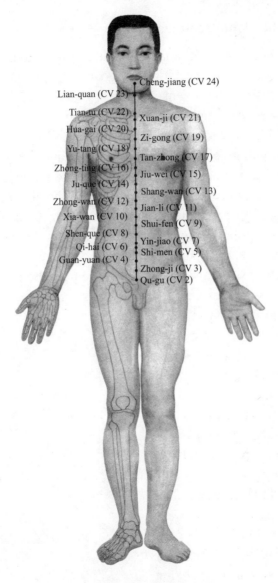

Cheng-jiang (CV 24)
Lian-quan (CV 23)
Tian-tu (CV 22)
Xuan-ji (CV 21)
Hua-gai (CV 20)
Zi-gong (CV 19)
Yu-tang (CV 18)
Tan-zhong (CV 17)
Zhong-ting (CV 16)
Jiu-wei (CV 15)
Ju-que (CV 14)
Shang-wan (CV 13)
Zhong-wan (CV 12)
Jian-li (CV 11)
Xia-wan (CV 10)
Shui-fen (CV 9)
Shen-que (CV 8)
Yin-jiao (CV 7)
Qi-hai (CV 6)
Shi-men (CV 5)
Guan-yuan (CV 4)
Zhong-ji (CV 3)
Qu-gu (CV 2)

Figure 3-41 (the conception vessel)

67

lower back pain.

Prevention And treatment

Once upon a time, in great knight's stories, to completely open up the conception and governor vessels was the way to realize the dream of eternal youthful life and endless power. Although that was just a fairy tale, a healthy and unblocked conception vessel does slow the aging process and will give you a lot more strength and vitality.

- One of the best and also convenient ways to take care of the conception vessel is pushing the abdomen. Using both hands, press and push downwards from the chest to underneath the belly button. You can add pressure gradually. Do this for 5 minutes every day before sleep and even better once more before getting up in the morning. It also relieves constipation.

- The Guan-yuan point is 3 Cuns below the belly button (Figure 3-42). It is where males store essence and females save blood. It is one of the key well-being points and can supply original energy and kidney energy. This is the number one well-being point for strong sexuality. The best way to stimulate this point is moxibustion (see

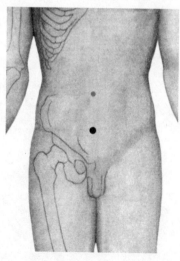

Figure 3-42 (the Guan-yuan point - CV 4)

Chapter 2) and best season to do so is winter. Massaging this area by pressing and rubbing with the hands is also very helpful.

- The Qi-hai point is 1.5 Cun below the belly button (Figure 3-43). It means the sea of energy in Chinese language. Frequently stimulating this point can summon up energy and make you full of life. Moxibustion and massage are effective

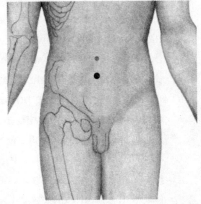

Figure 3-43 (the Qi-hai point - CV 6)

for this point. Abdominal breathing will bring oxygen deep into the lower abdomen and arouse energy in the Qi-hai point. Stand and relax your abdomen, and gently press the Qi-hai point; inhale deeply to bring the lower abdomen up; stop for a few seconds, and then exhale slowly and completely. Repeat this motion for several minutes. Some prefer doing it quickly when exhaling, this also works.

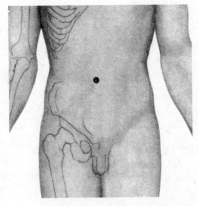

- The Shen-que point is in the middle of the belly button (Figure 3-44). It is also a key wellbeing point. There are several ways of

Figure 3-44 (the Shen-que point - CV 8)

69

taking care of it, but a needle cannot be used. Moxi-bustion is good, but the easiest way is just to press on it 100 times every day before sleep. The pressure used should be based on the person's comfort level, not too hard and not too gently. Before long, you will have better sleep, increased libido, and have more energy during the day. Remember, to have best results, when pressing the shen-que point, concentrate on the pressing and do the pressing with a good rhythm.

- The Tan-zhong point is the midpoint between the centers of the breasts (or the midpoint of the two nipples) (Figure 3-45). This is a soothing point. If you can't let out sad or burdensome feelings, massaging this point gives you great relief. It also heals coughs and chest congestion. This point can prevent many breast diseases and make the breasts look fuller and even.

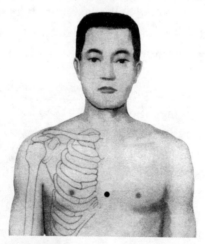

Figure 3-45 (the Tan-zhong point - CV 17)

14. The Governor Vessel – Where The Body's Yang Energy Rises

Introduction

The governor vessel is also one of the extraordinary meridians and does not belong to a particular organ. It is on the centerline of the upper body on the back side. It governs and adjusts the energy in all the Yang meridians. It runs through the spine and brain and inside connects to the kidneys, heart, and uterus. Therefore, the governor vessel is closely related to our mind, emotions, and sexuality.

As shown on figure 3-46, it starts from the inside the lower abdomen (if female, starts from the uterus), comes out from the perineum, along the center of the spine goes up and into the brain; it arrives at the top of the head, then drops down to the forehead, along the nose to the upper teeth; then it travels down to meet with the conception and Chong vessels. It also connects to the heart and kidneys.

There are total 28 acupuncture points on the governor vessel.

Common Syndromes Related To The Governor Vessel

Back pain, a rigid spine, cervical neck pain, headache, fever, stroke, memory loss, sleeplessness, and arthritis.

Prevention And treatment

As we have said in our discussion of the conception vessel section, to open up the conception and governor vessels was once believed to be the road leading to eternal youthfulness and endless power. We now know there is no nev-

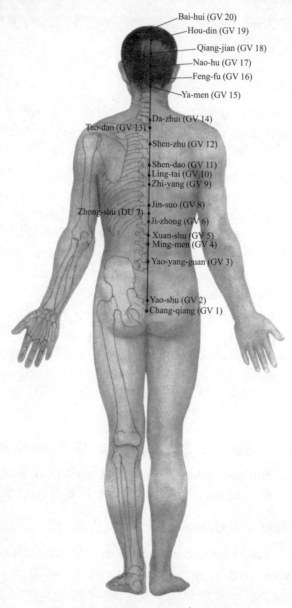

Figure 3-46 (the governor vessel)

er-ending life, but long and healthy living is certainly possible. Keeping the conception and governor vessels open and full of energy is one of the ways to achieve that goal.

- The Ming-men point is on the centerline of the back and at the same level as the bellybutton (Figure 3-47). This point can brace the lower back, and strengthen the kidneys and spleen functions. It cures back pain, enuresis (bedwetting), diarrhea, impotence, and premature ejaculation for men. It treats irregular menstruation and recurrent mis-carriages for women. Spend 3 minutes every day to warm this point by rubbing the area with the palms. You can thus strengthen the kidneys and spleen functions and increase your vitality.

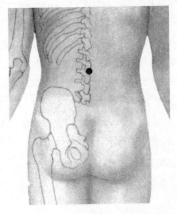

Figure 3-47
(the Ming-men point - GV 4)

- The Bai-hui point is the highest acupuncture point. It is on the top of the head and 5 Cuns behind the front hair line (Figure 3-48). It wakens the brain and raises the Yang energy. Pressing on this area with the palm in a circular movement and in a clockwise direction for 30 to 50 repetitions can clear your mind and lower blood pressure.

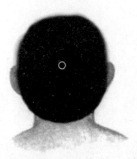

Figure 3-48
(the Bai-hui point - GV 20)

We have now discussed all 13 main meridians in detail. We live because we have lively organs. To live with great health, we need to have strong and vigorous organs, and the Jingluos are the pathways to supply energy and blood to them. Therefore, keeping the Jingluos in good shape and letting them stay open and efficient is the key to our over-all health and longevity.

From the preceding discussion, we can see that all the Yang meridians are located on the outer side of the body and all the Yin meridians are on the inner side. The organs that have Yin meridians are more vital, and therefore, they are placed at the inner side of the body and protected by the Yang meridians.

Our body has designed a brilliant system to support our lives, but it's important to learn how to make good use of them.

Chapter 4
Do-It-Yourself-Therapy For Disease Prevention And Common Syndrome Treatments

In this chapter, we will introduce the therapy methods that can target some of the diseases or symptoms that annoy tens of thousands of people around the world daily.

We mentioned in Chapter 1 that Chinese Medicine pays a tremendous amount of attention to disease prevention and treatment at the early stage of disease. This early attention is the goal of this chapter and this book. We don't want to wait until we are sick, even if we have the best treatment in the world. Being unwell is not a pleasant experience. We want to live every day with exuberance and cheerfulness, and thankfully, this goal is achievable. First, we need to understand the strengths and weaknesses of our bodies. Then we can take care of it directly and effectively. Second, spend time and effort to maintain your body (even your car needs regular maintenance and service!). Third, eat right and rest well. Lastly, keep positive in your thinking and do not to let negative issues bother you for too long.

The maintenance aspect of Chinese Medicine is what we are going to talk about in this chapter. When you maintain your body well, your body will make it much easier for you to have positive thinking. A person's ability to deal with emotional matters and tough situations is first of all a physical issue. A resilient body is the foundation for a happy and successful life, both physically and emotionally.

In the following sections, we present some of the therapy methods for specific diseases and symptoms. These methods are regularly practiced by some of the most accomplished Chinese Medicine doctors.

1. Common Cold

The common cold is the most common of all sicknesses. It is not fatal, but very bothersome. It is usually caused by invasion of cold air. It is better to take care of it in the beginning when you start to have colder then normal feelings, a stuffed nose, a tight and sore neck and back. Here is what to do:

- Knock or massage the large intestine meridians (Chapter 3, Section 2) for several minutes or until you feel less pain. You probably feel more pain now then in normal times.
- Massage the Feng-fu point and Feng-chi points for 3 to 5 minutes each. The Feng-fu point belongs to the governor vessel (Chapter 3, Section 14). It is on the center line of the neck on the back, the recess 1 Cun above the hairline is this point to massage (Figure 4-1). Keep this area warm even when you're not working on it.
- The Feng-chi points belong to the gallbladder meridians (Chapter 3 Section 11). They are next to and a little below the Feng-fu point in the low spots behind the ears and close to the hairline (Figure 4-2).
- The Da-zhui point: belongs to the governor vessel. It is on the center line of the neck on the back side. The low

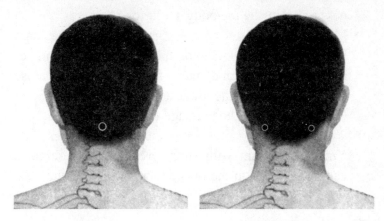

Figure 4-1
(the Feng-fu point - GV 16)

Figure 4-2
(the Feng-chi points - GB 20)

point below the seventh cervical vertebrae is the spot
for this point (Figure 4-3). Gently massage this point or
rub it with your palms to warm the area and let warm-

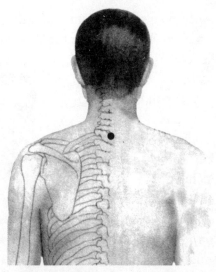

Figure 4-3 (the Da-zhui point - GV 14)

ness reach inside the body. Do it for 5 minutes.

- Massage the He-gu points. They belong to the large intestine meridians. One on the back of each hand between the thumb and index finger. When you close these two fingers, the highest point is the He-gu point (Figure 3-6). Do the massage for 3 minutes each.
- For a running nose and a stuffy nose, press the Ying-xiang point with some pressure for 2 minutes each time. It is on the outside and bottom of the nose wing (Figure 3-8).

2. Cough

The lung meridians (Chapter 3, Section 1) are the best cough medicines. If you get a cough easily, massaging the lung meridians should be a regular activity. In addition, all the acupuncture points on the lung meridians are good for easing a cough.

- The Yun-men points: are 6 Cuns from the vertical centerline of the upper body where the depressions underneath the collarbones lie (Figure 4-4).
- The Zhong-fu points are 1 Cun below the Yun-men points (Figure 4-4). They are the key points for curing bronchitis and asthma. Combining pressing and massaging Fei-shu points on the back will stop a cough very quickly (Figure 4-5).

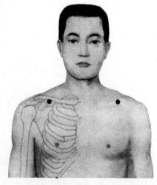

Figure 4-4
(the Yun-men point - LU 2)

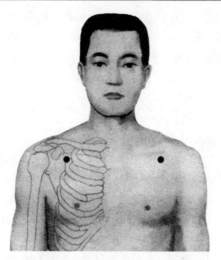

Figure 4-5 (the Zhong-fu point - LU 1)

- The Fei-shu points belong to the bladder meridians, 1.5 Cun from the vertical centerline of the back on the same level as the third thoracic vertebra (Figure 4-6).

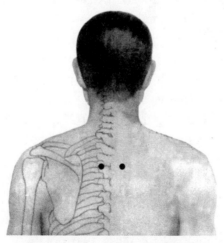

Figure 4-6 (the Fei-shu point - BL 13)

- Use the Chi-ze and Kong-zui points

  To find the Chi-ze point, bend the elbow. You'll find a tendon on the inner side of the arm. The point is in the recess inside the elbow on the thumb side of this tendon (Figure 3-3).

  The Kong-zui point is on the extension line of the index finger, 7 Cuns above the wrist line (Figure 3-4). Massaging these two points can heal a cough, breathing difficulty, chest pain, or a sore throat. These two points can be pressed harder to achieve better results.

- The Tai-yuan point is on the inner side of the wrist at the intersection of the wrist line and the extension line of the thumb where the pulse can be felt (Figure 3-2).

3. Asthma

The fundamental reason for having asthma is a weak immunity. It is caused by an invasion of external harmful forces through the mouth, nose and skin into the lungs. Therefore, the key to preventing asthma from coming back again and again is to protect and strengthen the lungs, supply them with enough energy and blood, which will prevents colds and allergy.

- Massage the lung meridians (Chapter 3, Section 1) to let the lungs have enough energy supply.
- Press and massage the He-gu points (Fgure 3-6) for 2 minutes each at least once a day. Massage the Fei-shu (Figure 4-6) points for 3 minutes daily, it would be better if you can also do cupping for 10 to 15 minutes (see Chapter 2) on these two points. This activates the positive energy inside the body.

- If asthma usually comes during spring and winter, that's due to offensive chilliness and cold air. Besides massaging the He-gu and Fei-shu points mentioned above, add the Zu-san-li points, also massage the Guan-yuan points and the Tai-xi points. These practices should be started before winter begins. When spring comes, massaging only the He-gu and Fei-shu points 200 times a day should be sufficient.

  The Zu-san-li points belong to the stomach meridians (Chapter 3 Section 3). There is a point on each leg and on the outer front side of the lower leg, measured 3 Cuns down from the bottom of the patella and right behind the tibia on the outer side (Figure 3-11). Press and massage each of the points 5 minutes daily. They are the number one wellbeing points, so massaging these two points can increase immune ability noticeably.

  The Guan-yuan point belongs to the conception vessel (Chapter 3 Section 13), 3 Cuns below the belly button (figure 3-42). The best way to use this point is through moxibustion, but if not available, pressing and massaging this point are also effective techniques. This point should be kept warm. Do the activity for 3 minutes daily.

  The Tai-xi points belong to the kidney meridians (Chapter 3 Section 8), and each is in the low spot behind the tip of the ankle bone (Figure 3-30). Massage each of these two points 3 minutes daily.

- If asthma easily comes during the summer, that's due to weak lungs plus heat and dampness inside the body. Therefore, besides the He-gu and Fei-shu points, we need to add the Zu-San-li points, the Yin-ling-quan points and the Yin-tang point. You need to start doing this activity before summer arrives.

Zu-san-li, (Figure 3-11), 3 to 5 minutes daily.

The Yin-ling-quan points belong to the spleen meridians (chapter 3 Section 4). Each one is located at the inner side of the lower leg with the low point at the upper end of the tibia (Figure 4-7). Do the massage for 3 to 5 minutes daily on each point.

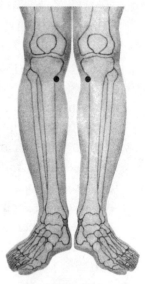

Figure 4-7
(the Yin-ling-quan points - SP 9)

The Yin-tang point: does not belong to any meridian. It is in between the eyebrows (Figure 4-8). Gently pinch it for 3 minutes daily.

- In addition, the Zhong-fu points (Figure 4-5) and the Yu-ji points, the Tai-yuan points (Figure 3-2) are commonly used for treating asthma as well. Try 3 to 5 minutes of massage on each of these points daily to see noticeable improvement.

The Yu-ji points belong to the lung meridians and are

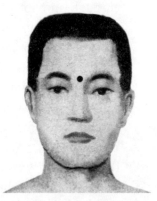

Figure 4-8 (the Yin-tang point)

inside of the palms on the thumb side, 1 Cun below the intersection lines between the thumbs and the palms (Figure 4-9).

4. Diabetes

Diabetes is a widespread disease and sacrifices the quality of life for many people. In Chinese Medicine theory, diabetes is caused by a deficiency of Yin energy.

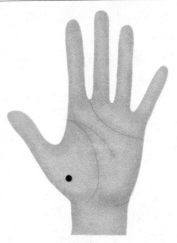

Figure 4-9 (the Yu-ji point - LU 10)

People who are most likely to have diabetes are those with a hyper stomach and those with fragile kidneys. Those with a hyper stomach eat a lot and easily become hungry. Those with fragile kidneys are generally weak and easily tire.

People with a hyper liver or a congested liver are also prone to diabetes. Hyper liver makes people easy to anger and a congested liver keeps you in low spirits and makes you feel upset.

A weak spleen (indigestion) can lead to diabetes too. The spleen is in charge of turning the food processed by the stomach into the energy that is later consumed by the entire body. A weak spleen will not be able to complete this task well. When sugar can not be converted into energy, it will stay in the blood, causing the diabetes.

Therefore, depend on the type of your physical condition and emphasize the related meridians that affect you the most. Frequently massaging these meridians will effectively reduce or let you avoid developing this annoying disease.

The following acupuncture points can help lower your blood sugar level:

- The San-yin-jiao points belong to the spleen meridians (Chapter 3 Section 4). Each is behind the tibia, 3 Cuns above the tip of the ankle bone (Figure 3-17).
- The Gong-sun points belong to the spleen meridians. They are on the inner sides of the feet, one on each foot and 1 Cun behind the big toe joint below the foot bones (Figure 3-16).
- The Tai-bai points are at the inner sides of the feet at the depressions behind and below the highest points of the toe joints (Figure 3-15).
- The Di-ji points belong to the spleen meridians. One is on each leg and 3 Cuns below the Yin-ling-quan point (Figure 4-7 and Figure 4-10.)

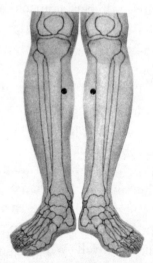

- The Fu-liu points belong to the kidney meridians (Chapter 3 Section 8). They are on the inner sides of the lower legs, one on each side and 2 Cuns above the highest point of the ankle bone and in front of the Achilles tendon (heel tendon) (Figure 4-11).

Figure 4-10 (the Di-ji points - SP 8)

- The Tai-xi points: See Figure 3-30.

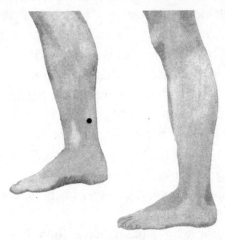

Figure 4-11 (the Fu-liu point - KI 7)

- The Yong-quan points belong to the kidney meridians. To find one, cover all the toes. The recess on the upper 1/3 line of the sole is this point (Figure 3-31).
- The Wan-gu points belong to the small intestine meridians (Chapter 3, Section 6). People with diabetes usually have dysfunctional small intestines. Wan-gu points are the primary points of the small intestine meridians (Figure 3-24). They have the strong ability to normalize the functions of the small intestine. Often massaging these points can help lower the glucose.

Massage each of these points for 3 to 5 minutes daily.

5. High Blood Pressure

- High blood pressure is also an epidemic disease that distresses many people in the US and around the world. It can lead to stroke, heart attack, heart failure, or kidney failure, and is a real "silent killer." In Chinese Medicine, the cause of high blood pressure is excessive Yang energy in the liver meridians (Chapter 3, Section 12) and a deficiency of Yin energy in the kidney meridians (Chapter 3, Section 8). By massaging the liver and kidney meridians regularly and massaging the He-gu points and Zu-san-li points as well, we can actually prevent high blood pressure.

The Hu-ge points belong to the large intestine medians (Figure 3-6).

The Zu-san-li point: belongs to the stomach meridians (Figure 3-11).

- For those who already have high blood pressure, there are still some simple things you can do. Press and massage the Tai-chong points, the Tai-xi points and the Qu-chi points for 3 to 5 minutes every day. Your blood pressure should be under control before long.

The Tai-chong points: belong to the liver meridians (Chapter 3, Section 12). Each is on the back of the foot between the big toe and the second toe. The recessed point between the highest point of the back and the end of the toe is where the point is (figure 3-40).

The Tai-xi points belong to the kidney meridians (Figure 3-30).

The Qu-chi points belong to the large intestine meridians (Chapter 3 Section 2), when you bend the elbows, the end points of the elbow line on the thumb sides, there are the Qu-chi points (Figure 3-7).

- The Yang-gu points can lower blood pressure too. These two points belong to the small intestine meridians (Chapter 3, Section 6), one on each hand. The dints in front of the wrist bones along the little fingers on the back of the hands are where these points are located (figure 4-12).

6. Breast Disease

Various types of breast disease trouble an enormous number of women every day around the world. Breast cancer is the most common form of cancer in women, and it is the number one or number two killer of women. The causes for breast diseases vary, but

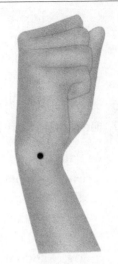

Figure 4-12
(the Yang-gu point - SI 5)

the ways to keep our breasts healthy are similar. First, we need to keep in good spirits, as a bad mood or depressed feeling make it hard for energy to move around in the liver meridians. Congested liver meridians cause breast disease, if congestion worsens badly, cancer occurs. Every lady should practice the following steps often to eliminate the hidden danger of breast disease and breast cancer.

- Frequently massage the liver meridians (Chapter 3, Section 12) and knock on the gallbladder meridians (Chapter 3, Section 11), no less then 10 minutes each time.
- Press and massage the Tai-chong points (Figure 3-40) 3 to 5 minutes every day.
- Press and massage the Tan-zhong point 3 minutes every day. This point belongs to the conception vessel (Chapter 3, Section 13). It is the mid-point between

the center of the breasts (or the mid-point between the two nipples) (Figure 3-45). This point can also soothe uneasy feelings and make the breasts look even and fuller. When massaging this point, do it in a clockwise direction or rub it downwardly.

7. Menstruation Problems

1) <u>Painful menstruation</u>:
Many women have the problem, and the cause can be different, so the treatment methods should also differ based on the causes.

- <u>Energy deficiency</u>: always lets one feel pain in the lower abdomen during or a few days after the period. It feels better if this area is pressed; this case also gives trouble sleeping and a small amount of bleeding in light color.

If this is your case, you need to gather more energy from the Qi-hai point and the Zu-san-li points.

The Qi-hai point is on the conception vessel (Chapter 3, Section 13), located 1.5 Cuns below the belly button (Figure 3-43). Abdomen breathing is the easiest way to gather energy from Qi-hai. Just put one hand on the point, slowly inhale with the nose, let the lower abdomen (instead of the chest) pump up, and exhale slowly with the mouth. At the same time gently push the Qi-hai point and deflate the abdomen completely. Repeat 10 to 20 times for a set, and do one set a day.

Press and massage the Zu-san-li points for 5 minutes a day, as they belong to the stomach meridians (Figure 3-11).

- Liver depression is pain and bloating in the lower abdomen, swelling and painful breasts, a dark color period with blood clots, low spirits, and habitual sighing.

  This is what to do for this case: starting one week before the period. Every day, knock on each side of the gallbladder meridians for 5 minutes first, and, before you go to bed, massage the Tai-chong points (Figure 3-40) and the Xue-hai points for 2 minutes each. The Xue-hai points (Figure 3-18) belong to the spleen meridians (Chapter 3 Section 4). Stop massaging the Xue-hai points when the period comes; otherwise too much bleeding might occur. If pain is severe, press the pain killer He-gu points (Figure 3-6).

2) Irregular menstruation:

- Early menstruation is when the period always comes early, some times more then a week early with light color. One always feels tired and often has a bloating stomach after a meal. This condition is because of the weak spleen. The spleen manages the blood circulation, and the blood can not be held well if the spleen is feeble. Therefore, the period comes early. To solve this problem, use the acupuncture points on the spleen and stomach meridians; three is sufficient. Use the Xue-hai points (Figure 3-18), the Zu-san-li points (Figure 3-11) and the San-yin-jiao points (Figure 3-17)

  Just 7 days before the period, massage each of these points for 3 minutes every day before going to bed at night. You can stop after the period comes.

- Prolonged menstruation is when the period lasts more

than ten days with a smaller amount and light colored bleeding. You can, feel faint sometimes as well as experience back and leg weakness. This condition is mostly caused by fragile kidneys, hence something needs to be done to support the kidneys. Three points are all you need to get help. Use: the Guan-yuan point, the Shen-shu points, and the Tai-xi points.

The Guan-yuan point belongs to the conception vessel (Chapter 3, Section 13), 3 Cuns below the belly-button (Figure 3-42). Using both bands, the right hand on top of the left hand, press and massage this point in a counter clockwise direction for 2 minutes every night before sleep.

The Shen-shu points belong to the bladder meridians (Chapter 3 Section 7) and are the kidney passage points. They are on the back 1.5 Cun from the center-line of the back vertically and right below the second lumbar vertebrae (Figure 4-13). Warm them up by

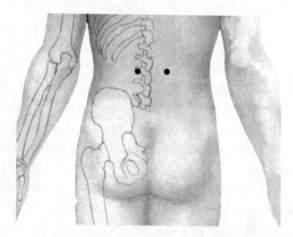

Figure 4-13 (the Shen-shu points - BL 23)

rubbing on the area with both hands for 1 minute every night before sleep.

The Tai-xi points, belong to the kidney meridians (Figure 3-30). Massage and press on them with the thumbs for 2 minutes every night before sleep.

Do these massages during your menstrual period.

- Early menstruation with emotional upset. Here the period comes quite early, and before it comes, the breasts and lower abdomen swell and are painful. You also experience low spirits, a bad mood, and irritability. In this case, you need to control the blood and ease the liver by massaging the Xue-hai points, the Tai-chong points and the Xing-jian points.

The Xue-hai points (Figure 3-18).

The Tai-chong points (Figure 3-40).

The Xing-jian points belong to the liver meridians (Chapter 3, Section 12), one on each foot, are in front of the Tai-chong point and at the root of the toes (Figure 4-14)

During the period, press and massage each of these three points on both sides for 2 minutes every night before sleep. Massage the Tai-chong points whenever you have a bad mood.

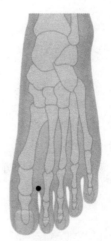

Figure 4-14
(the Xing-jian point - LR 2)

- Late period or a small amount bleeding. Massage the Shui-quan and Jiao-xin points. They belong to the kidney meridians.

The Shui-quan points are 1 Cun directly below the Tai-xi points (Figure 3-30) where the lowest points behind the ankle bones are located (Figure 4-15).

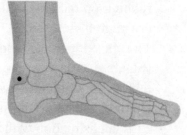

Figure 4-15 (the Shui-quan point - KI 5)

The Jiao-xin points are 2 Cuns above the Tai-xi points and 0.5 Cuns closer to the tibia bone (Figure 4-16).

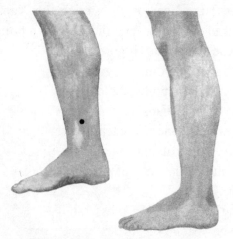

Figure 4-16 (the Jiao-xin point - KI 8)

8. Overweight

Overweight is not just a problem any more, it is an epidemic around the globe. There are so many people trying different ways to solve it, including exercise, diet, pills and more. Some work, and most don't. When we are busy spending so much money and effort to look into numerous options everywhere, do we think that the solution might just be within ourselves? In this section, we'll look at the weight problem from the Chinese Medicine point of view and try to make sense of it by analyzing how our bodies work and fail to work. Therefore, we might find the solution for this unpleasant and frustrating situation.

The reasons for overweight vary, so the solutions are also different.

1) Most overweight people overeat; overeating overworks the stomach and spleen. Their functions weaken because of exhaustion, and they have no power to digest the food and move energy and blood. Fat accumulation happens. This situation should be dealt with by improving the functionalities of the stomach and spleen using the following methods:

- Knock the stomach meridians and massage the spleen meridians (Chapter 3, section 3 & 4) everyday for 10 to 15 minutes each. If you always have stomach bloating after meals (sometimes in the afternoon even without a meal), or drool while sleeping, your spleen is not working well. Massaging the spleen meridians is a must, especially the portions on the lower legs (inner side, along the tibia). You probably feel more pain in these areas, but keep doing it to unclog the meridian congestion.
- Press and massage the Zu-san-li points (Figure 3-11).
- Press and massage the Tian-shu points and the Zhong-wan point for 3 minutes each between half an hour and one hour after dinner every day. Also massage the lower abdomen (clock wise) for 3 minutes. TheTian-shu points belong to the stomach meridians and are on the

same level with the belly button and 2 Cuns from it vertically (Figure 3-12). The Zhong-wan point belongs to the conception vessel on the centerline of the front body, 4 Cuns above the belly button (Figure 4-17).

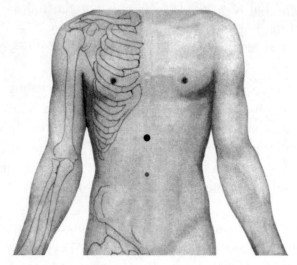

Figure 4-17 (the Zhong-wan point - CV12)

This procedure is also very good for healing chronic stomach problems.

- Knee-walking, Yes, do walk on your knees! A very effective and fast way to drive energy and blood down to the lower body and the knee areas. During the process, built-up fat is flushed away. Just put a comfortable mat on the floor, and start to walk on the knees. If the knees hurt or you have knee problems, use more cushions and walk slowly or don't walk in the beginning. If you can knee-walk for 20 minutes daily, you will be pleased with the result in 2 to 3 weeks, especially around the thigh areas.

- This method is also great for treating knee problems, back problems, some times even hair loss. Don't knee walk immediately after meals. This is the time when the stomach needs both energy and blood the most to process the food just eaten. Knee walking will quickly attract energy and blood to the knees, which will affect the work of the stomach.

2) Liver and gallbladder dysfunction or under function can cause weight gain. As we discussed in last chapter, the liver removes the toxins from the blood and the gallbladder receives bile from the liver and then releases it to digest food, and break down fat and cholesterols whenever needed. If the liver performs poorly, the detoxification procedure is impaired, and not enough bile is produced. Therefore, digestion is not complete, waste cannot be eliminated from the body, and the result is accumulation of useless fat, especially round the thighs and on both sides of the waist (the love handles). To deal with this issue, use the following methods.

- To clean up fat on the inner side of the thighs, massage the liver meridians (Chapter 3, Section 12) by pressing and pushing on them from the root of the thighs to the knees, You can use some lotion as a lubricator. Repeat 300 times every night before sleep.
- To clean up the fat on the outer side of the thighs, knock on the gallbladder meridians (Chapter 3, section 11), from the outer sides of the hips all the way to the knees. Do it for 5 to 10 minutes on each side.
- To clean up the fat on the waist, knock the belt vessel. Use your fists to pound the sides of the waist 300 times while lying on the back, add force gradually,

do not exceed your comfort level.

3) When the bladder meridians (Chapter 3, section 7) are not working properly, fat usually accumulates on the back, hips, and back of the legs because the bladder meridians run on the back of the body. Unclogging these meridians is the key task. Since they are on the back, some help from family members may be needed. Massage along the meridians, back-pinching (see Chapter 3, Section 7 and Figure 3-28 for how), knock on the hips and back of the legs frequently.

Other methods can also be used as we mentioned in Chapter 2, such as cupping (sucking a vacuumed cup onto the skin), scraping (scratching the skin with massage oil and a piece of thin plank made of cattle horn), to draw the coldness and dampness from inside of the body. It slows down circulation of the energy and blood.

4) Other meridian blockage can cause weight gain for the same reason that sluggish energy and blood flow will leave waste inside the body, making people fat and also sick. If the small intestine and heart meridians don't function well, you'll find the inner sides of the arms soft and floppy. This condition is a reminder to massage your small intestine meridians (Chapter 2, Section 6) and the heart meridians (Chapter 3, Section 5). It not only reduces the fat deposits, but also strengthens the organ functions. Massaging the large intestine meridians (Chapter 3, Section 2) can reduce the fat on the outer sides of the arms, and also relieves constipation caused by the lazy large intestine.

5) If any thing is accumulated, that's because the output amount is smaller then the input amount, and so is the fat in the body. The slow metabolism causes low energy us-

age, if the food intake is not also low, the energy will be stored in the body in the form of fat. Therefore, if we can increase our metabolism rate, it means less or no fat will build up and higher energy level. A simple abdomen breath can do that: Stand and relax your abdomen. Then gently press the Qi-hai point (Figure 3-43), inhale deeply with the nose to bring the lower abdomen up; stop for a few seconds, and then exhale through the mouth slowly (or quickly) and completely. Do this exercise for 5 to 10 minutes whenever you need energy instead of eating junk food. Do not do the abdomen breathing immediately after meals.

6) Finally, nothing will work well if you just hold on to unhealthy habits, such as always eating junk food or simply overeating anything, never exercise, always stay up late and not get enough sleep. When we understand more about our bodies, we realize that damage control should be done before damage happens.

From the above discussion, we can see that losing weight is not an isolated issue. It is about normalizing the entire body's functionalities, it is about the wellbeing of the whole of our lives. You have to love yourself enough to take positive actions and stop negative ones.

9. Constipation

Constipation is another widespread problem in modern society. If the body cannot get rid of the waste and toxics periodically, they will stay there. When there is more and more waste in the body, all sorts of bad things happen. Something can be done at home by yourself to eliminate this annoyance.

• Massage each of the Tian-shu points (Figure 3-12) for

3 minutes before bed and before getting up in the morning followed by massaging the lower abdomen for 2 to 3 minutes using both hands (clockwise). Doing so can increase the peristaltic movement of the large intestine and break up the feces inside for easier excretion. This is a very effective way to relieve constipation.

- Press the He-gu (Figure 3-6) points with both hands with some force and with your mind concentrating on the pressing for a few minutes. This action will move the large intestine, and a lot of times, bring you an immediate result.

- Abdomen pushing and belt vessel knocking. Lying on the bed, using both hands, press on the abdomen and slide down from the chest all the way down below the belly button. Do it for 5 minutes each time. The belt vessel is around the waistline, so lying on the bed and using both fists, knock on both sides of the waist (the love handles) 300 times. The pressure and force used should be added little by little, always based on your personal comfort level. Do these actions once in the night and once in the morning.

- Often knocking on the large intestine meridians (Chapter 3, Section 2) is good for helping the movement of the large intestine and lessens the chance of constipation. The Shang-yang points are at the top of the index fingers, right next to the end of the nails on the thumb sides (Figure 4-18).These points can act like laxatives in case you feel feces coming, but just can't get them out, so pressing these two points will open up the lock just like the He-gu points we talked about above will do.

- Drink a lot of warm water, not icy cold water, because coldness slows down energy and blood. Two glasses of warm water right after getting up in the morning will do a good job of flushing the large intestine.

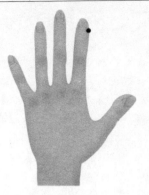

Figure 4-18
(the Shang-yang point - LI 1)

10. Irritability

Seldom having a good mood, feeling tight in the chest, and being easy to get angry is mostly because of a congested liver. Hospital check-ups probably will say nothing is wrong, but you can make yourself feel better by simply doing the following:

Take a foot bath (a fantastic way to free up energy and blood flows in all meridians) for half hour in the evening, followed by massaging the Tai-chong (Figure 3-40) and the Xing-jian (Figure 4-14) points by pressing on the Tai-chong point and pushing down to the Xing-jian point in one direction. Use some lotion for easier movement. Repeat for 3 minutes on both feet. Do it every day.

11. Depression

Today, stresses can come from anywhere and can be about anything. There is no way that we can avoid stressful situations as long as we live in this modern society. Knowing we can't change the world, we have to make ourselves more sustainable to the foreign influences. In the heart meridian section (Chapter 3, Section 5), we pointed out that

for cardiovascular health.

- To prevent angina, you can press and massage the Xi-men points. They are on the pericardium meridians, one on each arm and 5 Cuns above the wrist line (Figure 4-20). You can put more pressure on the Xi-men points because they are deeper.

  If angina strikes, take your medicine and also press and massage these points (especially the left one) to relieve the pain more quickly. If you have coronary heart disease, you should press the Xi-men points and the ji-quan points (Figure 3-21) every day for several minutes. In addition, the Zhong-fu points are good for preventing angina (Figure 4-5).

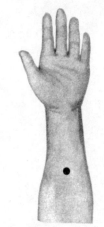

Figure 4-20
(the Xi-men point - PC 4)

13. Sleeplessness

If you have trouble sleeping, you know how precious a good night sleep is. There are so many people disturbed by sleeplessness. The causes can be different, but mostly, they all relate to uneasiness of the heart, mind, or liver. There are things you can do to get your sleep back and be fully recharged for the next day.

- If you always wake up around 1 or 2 o'clock in the early morning and it is difficult to get back to sleep, there is excessive hotness in your liver. Massaging the liver meridians (Chapter 3, Section 12) and the Tai-chong points (Figure 3-40) is what you should do before you go to bed at night to let out the fire. When massaging the liver meridians, you can press and push from the bottom of the thighs (inner sides) all the way down to the lower legs. Use some lotion for comfort. Do this for 5 to 10 minutes each leg, and then massage the Tai-chong points for 3 to 5 minutes each side.

- For people who just have a hard time falling into sleep or seldom have high quality sleep, the following suggestions will help:

The Shen-men points: belong to the heart meridians (Chapter 3, Section 5). When you bend your fist inward, you'll find a hard tendon on the little finger side. The intersection between the wrist line and this tendon is the Shen-men point, one on each hand (Figure 3-20). These points calm the heart and clear the mind, so 3 minutes massage on each point each time is sufficient.

The Da-ling points: belong to the pericardium meridians (Chapter 3, Section 9). They are located at the midpoint of the wrist lines (Figure 3-33). Massage each point for 3 minutes each time.

The Bai-hui point: belongs to the governor vessel, it is on the top of the head 5 Cuns behind the front hairline on the centerline of the head (Figure 3-48). Sit straight, use one palm press on this point and massage, every 10 circles adds one vertical vibration (pat with hand). Repeat for 10 minutes every day.

- A foot bath for 30 minutes every night before sleep will relax you and bring you to sleep nicely. Use the hottest water you can comfortably tolerate.

like. These could be because of a dysfunctional stomach or spleen or both. Generally, if you have an appetite, but don't feel comfortable after eating, that's a stomach problem. If your appetite is not good and the food doesn't get digested after eating, that's a spleen problem.

Knock and massage each side of the stomach meridians (Chapter 3, Section 3) for 10 to 15 minutes every day. Press and massage each of the Zu-san-li points for 5 minutes every day and develop sensible eating habits, then you will find yourself never needing to worry about stomach problems.

1) Stomach problems can be dealt with by using the Zu-san-li points and the Tian-shu points.

The Zu-san-li points belong to the stomach meridians, and they are the number one wellbeing points (Figure 3-11).

The Tian-shu points belong to the stomach meridians, (see Figure 3-12 for their locations).

Press and massage these points for 3 to 5 minutes every day to normalize stomach functions.

2) Spleen problems can be treated by massaging the spleen meridians (Chapter 3, Section 4) specially the parts on the lower legs. Also massage the Zu-san-li points and the Pi-shu points.

For the Zu-san-li points, see Figure 3-11.

The Pi-shu points: belong to the bladder meridians (Chapter 3, Section 7), and they are the passage points of the spleen. They are 1.5 Cun vertically from the centerline of the back on each side and right below the 11th thoracic vertebrae (Figure 4-21).

Press and massage each of the Zu-san-li points for 3

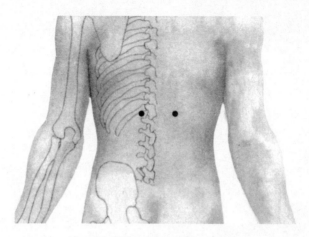

Figure 4-21 (the Pi-shu point - BL 20)

minutes after a meal. Massage the Pi-shu points for 3 to 5 minutes, do this one hour before bedtime. You will need some help from other people. If you can, do cupping for 15 minutes on the Pi-shu points every other day. That will be more effective.

3) For bloating or vomiting: use the Zu-san-li and Zhong-wan points and abdomen pushing.

For the Zu-san-li points. see Figure 3-11.

The Zhong-wan points: belong to the conception vessel (see Figure 4-17).

For Abdomen pushing, see the constipation section of this chapter.

For half an hour after meals, press and massage the Zhong-wan point for 5 minutes and the Zu-san-li points for 3 minutes each. Do abdomen pushing 100 times before bedtime and again before getting up in the morning.

It is always important not to eat too much at one meal and to chew all food thoroughly before swallowing.

the small intestine meridians and are located at the back of the forearms 5 Cuns above the wrist lines and on the extension line of the little fingers (Figure 4-25).

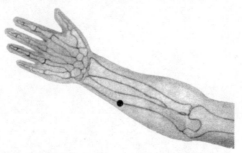

Figure 4-25 (the Zhi-zheng point - SI 7)

Massage the small intestine meridians especially on the portions of the hands and forearms, as most of the points here deal with headaches. If you find any points are more painful when pressed, massage them more.

17. Migraine

- Do the same as described in the first part of Section 16 on 'headaches' in this chapter.
- Press and massage the Tian-chi points and the Tan-zhong points for 5 minutes.
  The Tian-chi points belong to the pericardium meridians (Chapter 3, Section 9). See Figure 4-19.
- The Tan-zhong point belongs to the conception vessel (Chapter 3, Section 13). See Figure 3-45.
- Knock along the stomach meridians (Chapter 3 Section 3).

18. Foggy Mind

Some times when you have a foggy mind, you just can't think straight. It may be due to lack of sleep or some other reason. Here are some simple ways to clear the mind and let you concentrate on what you are doing.

- Press and massage the Bai-hui point on the top of the head (Figure 3-48). It belongs to the governor vessel (Chapter 3, Section 14). Press on it with some pressure and massage for several minutes whenever needed.

- Hands crossing helps too. Close the right and left hands with ten fingers crossing each other, squeeze tightly for 3 seconds, relax, and switch the finger crossing positions and squeeze again (Figure 4-26). This equals one round, so repeat for several rounds each time. This action will stimulate the brain and make it more alert.

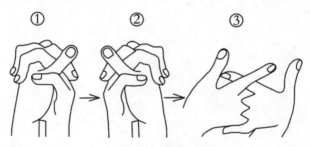

Figure 4-26 (hands crossing)

- Hands clapping is helpful. Stretch the both arms upwards and clap both hands with some force 3 times and then stretch the arms straight forward and clap 3 times (Figure 4-27).The sound sends a strong signal

111

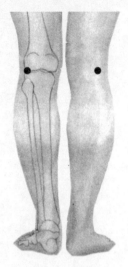 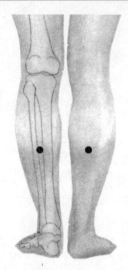

Figure 4-30
(the Wei-yang points - BL 39)

Figure 4-31
(the Cheng-shan points - BL 57)

lower legs, the muscles form a 'V' shape. The low point at the bottom tip of the 'V' is this point and is the same on the other leg (Figure 4-31).

To find one of the Fei-yang points, locate the mid-point between the ankle and the knee joint. Go 1 Cun down. This is the horizontal line; draw a vertical line from the back of the knee and move 1.5 Cun back. the intersection between the horizontal and vertical lines is the Fei-yang point. There is one on each leg. These points are especially effective for chronic back pain (stressed lumbar muscles). See Figure 4-32.

Press and massage each of these points for 4 minutes at a time.

Rub to warm the Shen-shu points and Ming-men point on the back. The Shen-shu points belong to the bladder meridians (Figure 4-13) and the Ming-men point belongs to the governor vessel (Figure 3-47). These three points are on the same level, therefore you can rub them at the same time. Do it for 3 to 5 minutes daily.

20. Cervical Neck Pain

Neck pain or cervical neck pain is no longer a disease only for older people. More and more, younger people develop this problem because of the way we are living and working. Long hours of sitting in front of computers and desks without proper exercise is the major

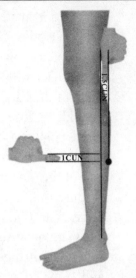

Figure 4-32
(the Fei-yang point - BL 58)

cause. In the beginning, the neck and shoulders are just sore and stiff , and then it becomes more painful and serious with difficulty turning the neck, numbness in the hands. Not enough blood is being supplied to the brain, causing dizziness and a foggy mind. Here we have some methods to prevent it, or relieve and stop the suffering.

- Knock and massage the three Yang meridians on the arms. These are large intestine meridians (Chapter 3, Section 2), the Sanjiao meridians (Chapter 3, Section 10) and the small intestine meridians (Chapter 3, section 6) for several minutes daily.
- Press and massage the Tian-zong points for 1 or 2 minutes each. The Tian-zong points belong to the small intestine meridians and are a little above the center points of the shoulder blades, parallel to the

115

fourth dorsal vertebra (Figure 3-25). These are very sensitive points, so you'll know when you find them.

- The Hou-xi points belong to the small intestine meridians (chapter 3, Section 6), and they are located on the back of the hands on the little finger sides. Close one hand. There is a line pointed to the tip of the little finger; the depression behind the end of this line is the Hou-xi point (Figure 4-33). The Hou-xi points are easy to find and easy to reach. They are great for normalizing the functions of the cervical vertebra and spine. If you are working in front of a desk, just roll your hands on the desk with the Hou-xi points underneath for 3-5 minutes every hour. It will relieve and prevent t neck pain very effectively.

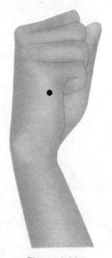

Figure 4-33
(the Hou-xi point - SI 3)

- Stretch the chest by raising both arms (with the forearms bent) to the same level as the shoulders and move backwards to squeeze the back and return. Repeat for 1 or 2 minutes whenever needed.
- Do some back pinching: See 'lower back pains' in this chapter.

21. Knee Problems

Many people over 40 have some of kind of knee problems. Most are due to degeneration of the joints. When less and less energy and blood can travel down to the knee areas, more and more serious will the problems become.

Our goal is to activate the positive energy and bring it down to the knees along with fresh blood.

- The 5 points to massage: the Xue-hai points, the Yin-ling-quan points, the Zu-san-li points, the Liang-qiu points and the Yang-ling-quan points.

  the Xue-hai points belong to the spleen meridians (Chapter 3, Section 4). See Figure 3-18.

  the Yin-ling-quan points: belong to the spleen meridians (Figure 4-7).

  For the Zu-san-li points, see Figure 3-11.

  The Liang-qiu points: belong to the stomach meridians (Chapter 3 section 3). They are on the front of the leg, 2 Cuns above the upper edge of the knee caps. These points can be applied using more force (Figure 4-34).

  The Yang-ling-quan points belong to the gallbladder meridians (Chapter 3, Section 11). They are on the outer

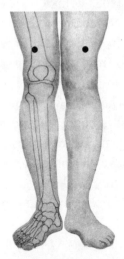

Figure 4-34
(the Liang-qiu points - ST 34)

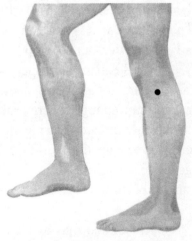

Figure 4-35
(the Yang-ling-quan point-GB 34)

117

sides of the legs 1 Cun below the bottom of the knee joints. The depressions a little in front of the round bones are the Yang-ling-quan points (Figure 4-35).

Press and massage these points 3 to 5 minutes each day, and rub the knees with the hands for 3 minutes daily to warm these areas for better blood circulation. Do it with some pressure.

- Knee walk for 10 to 20 minutes every day (see 'over-weight' section of this chapter). If your knees hurt, use more cushions or just kneel on the mat without walking in the beginning. After a while you'll be able to walk on your knees with comfort.

22. Beauty Matters

We all want to keep a youthful looking face for as long as we can. As we get older, the color of the face becomes dull and the youthful glow starts to fade, wrinkles appear here and there, eye bags start to appear, face muscles loosen and there is less shine in the eyes. Even the most expensive cosmetics can not stop the process from happening.

All these changes happen because the Jingluos (the meridians) are not as open as they were when we were younger, and not enough energy and blood is being transported to the face area. Knowing this problem, the main task is clear. Open up the meridians and make the body able to generate a sufficient amount of energy and blood and smoothly dispatch both everywhere in need, including our face.

1) Knock and massage the stomach meridians (chapter 3, Section 3) from underneath the neck all the way down to the feet every day. The majority of energy and blood sup-

ply on the face is provided by the stomach meridians; there-fore, keeping them open keeps the face with good energy and blood. You will have a naturally glowing look and re-silient skin. The large intestine meridians (Chapter 3, Sec-tion 2) also control some of the energy and blood passages to the face, so you should knock on these meridians on the arms every day as well.

2) Dark eyes and Eye Bags.

- Dark eyes are the result of congested and deficient en-ergy and blood in the liver, and often happen after too little sleep. Therefore, the target is to supply the liver with more energy and blood. Use four points to fulfill this purpose -- the Ge-shu points, the Gan-shu points, the San-yin-jiao points and the Tai-xi points.

  Knocking on the gallbladder meridians is an excel-lent way to decongest both the gallbladder and the liv-er meridians. Use your fists to pound on the outer sides of the legs and especially the upper portions, starting from the sides of the hips. Knock them every night for 5 to 10 minutes before going to bed.

  The Ge-shu points belong to the bladder meridians (Chapter 3, Section 7). They are the passage points of the diaphragm. They are located on the back 1.5 Cun from the centerline of the back vertically and right un-derneath the 7th thoracic vertebrae (Figure 4-36).

  The Gan-shu points also belong to the bladder meridi-ans. They are the passage points of the liver 1.5 Cun from the centerline of the back vertically and right un-derneath the 9th thoracic vertebrae (Figure 4-37).

  The San-yin-jiao points:belong to the spleen meridians
    See Figure 3-17.

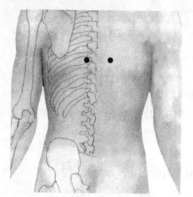 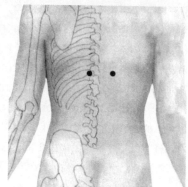

Figure 4-36
(the Ge-shu points - BL 17)

Figure 4-37
(the Gan-shu points - BL 18)

The Tai-xi points: belong to the kidney meridians.
See Figure 3-30.

Before going to bed every night, press and massage the
Ge-shu, Gan-shu and Tai-xi points for 3 to 5 minutes
each and the San-yin-jiao points for 3 minutes each.
Since the Ge-shu and Gan-shu points are on the back,
some help from other people will be needed.

- Eye bags are caused by the body's lowered ability to
  eliminate excessive water. Therefore, reactivating this
  ability is our approach to get rid of ugly eye bags. Three
  points are used, the Zu-san-li points, the Shui-fen point
  and the Yin-ling-quan points.

The Zu-san-li points are the number one well being
points and belong to the stomach meridians (Figure
3-11).

The Yin-ling-quan points: belong to the spleen meridians. See Figure 4-7 for locations.

The Shui-fen point belongs to the conception vessel
(Chapter 3. Section 13) and is 1 Cun above the belly

button on the front centerline of the body.

This is a very good point for normalizing the water deposit in the body (Figure 4-38). Every night before going to bed, press and massage these three points for 3 to 5 minutes each. If you can

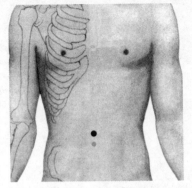

Figure 4-38 (the Shui-fen point - CV 9)

do moxibustion on the Zu-san-li and Shui-fen points, the result will be even better.

- Massaging the Cuan-zu points, the Jing-ming points and the Si-bai points will also help reduce dark eyes and eye bags.

The Cuan-zhu points belong to the bladder meridians (Chapter 3, Section 7). They are the little dents at the ends of the eyebrows on the inner sides of the eyes (Figure 4-39). The Jing-ming points

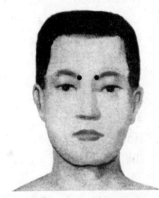

Figure 4-39 (the Cuan-zhu points - BL 2)

belong to the bladder meridians. The little dents a bit above the inner corners of the eyes are where they are located. (Figure 4-40).

The Si-bai points belong to the stomach meridians. They are below the pupils when looking straight ahead.

121

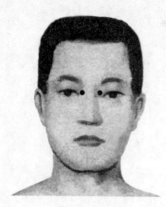 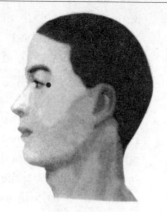

Figure 4-40
(the Jing-ming points - BL 1)

Figure 4-41
(the Tong-zi-liao point - GB 1)

The little dent on the cheekbones are the Si-bai points (Figure 3-13).

For wrinkles, besides knocking and massaging the stomach and large intestine meridians as described already, the following points can offer further help.

To prevent and reduce wrinkles around eyes, besides knocking on the gallbladder meridians, massage the Tong-zi-liao points and the Si-zhu-kong points.

The Tong-zi-liao points belong to the gallbladder meridians, 0.5 Cun from the outer corner of the eyes where the depressions are (Figure 4-41).

The Si-zhu-kong point: belong to the Sanjiao meridians (Chapter 3, Section 10). They are the little dents just below the outer ends of the eyebrows (figure 4-42).

There are many acupuncture points around the eyes, and a good way to massage them is to use the sides of your index fingers to scrape the edge of the orbital bones on both sides. This will maintain good eyesight if you do it regularly.

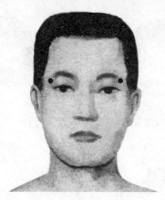

Figure 4-42 (the Si-zhu-kong points - TE 23)

- To prevent and reduce wrinkles on the face, use the Quan-liao points, the Ju-liao points, the Si-bai points and the Ren-ying points. These points are all great for blood circulations on the face and will keep the muscles and skin tight and resilient.

The Quan-liao points belong to the small intestine meridians (Chapter 3, Section 6) are the dents below the cheekbones and on the vertical line of the outer ends of the eyes (Figure 4-43).

The Ju-liao points belong to the stomach meridians below the center of the eyes and on the same level as the bottom of the nose (Figure 4-44).

For the Si-bai points, see Figure 3-13.

The Ren-ying points belong to the stom-

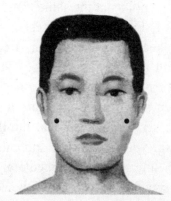

Figure 4-43 (the Quan-liao points - SI 18)

123

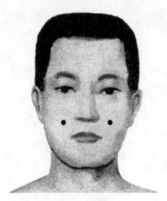 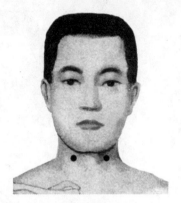

Figure 4-44
(the Ju-liao points - ST 3)

Figure 4-45
(the Ren-ying points - ST 9)

ach meridians on the front side of the neck, 1.5 Cun from the center and at the same level with the Adam's apple where the pulse can be felt (Figure 4-45). You will cough if you push too hard on these points. Just gently press on them or rub the area vertically with the rhythm of your inhaling and exhaling.

Gently massage the entire face mostly in an upward direction. In this way, you are massaging many points at the same time.

4) Finally, we'll present a simple and effective method to keep your face clear, free of spots and wrinkles, and with a youthful radiance. This method comes from a famous book written by one of the imperial doctors more then seven hundred years ago and originally was just for the service of the royal families: every night before sleep, calm your heart first and rub both your palms more then 10 times. Then immediately cover your face with the warmed hands for a few seconds. When you feel less warm, with your hands still pressing on the face, gently

start to massage the face in a circular motion. Do not rub the face, but repeat this procedure three or more times.

As you already know, there are six Yang meridians going through our face. By doing the face warming method above, we activate the energy inside these meridians. Also there are three Yin meridians going through each of our hands, Yin and yang energy are balanced with the transmission of warmth between the hands and face. You see, sometimes, the simplest thing has the most profound meaning.

23. Eye Protection

It is easy to take eyesight for granted when you have a good pair of eyes and perfect vision, but problems like near-sightedness, far-sightedness, glaucoma, cataract sand other vision or eye disorders trouble many people every day. These problems could come to you too if care is not taken. Let's protect our eyes, let them stay bright and lively, so we can always see clearly. These are the points you should massage everyday to stay away from eye problems. They are all on the face and around the eyes. They are the Jing-ming points (Figure 4-40), the Cuan-zhu points (Figure 4-39), the Si-bai points (Figure 3-13), the Cheng-qi points, the Tai-yang points (Figure 4-22) and the Yin-tang point (Figure 4-8).

The Cheng-qi points belong to the stomach meridians (Chapter 3, Section 3) and are below the pupils when looking straight ahead and on the edge of the orbital bones (Figure 4-46).

Sit or lie on your back, and then press and massage these points for 3 minutes each. Do not use too much pressure. Press only until it feels a little sore. Also, relax the eyes at least every hour when you are reading or working on computers.

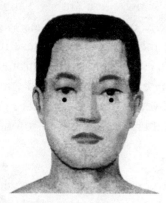

Figure 4-46 (the Cheng-qi points - St 1)

We have listed prevention and treatment methods for 23 common diseases or situations in the above sections. There are more then one method presented here for most of the cases. You can pick the ones that fit you the most.

Chapter 5
The Wisdom Of Wellbeing

We have nothing without health. A healthy body is the foundation of all other matters in life. A healthy body supports a sharp mind, clear thinking, good judgment, and balances the emotions.

Sometimes it is too late to realize that truth, and a lot of times we learn it in a hard way we did not expect. A wise person learns from somebody else's experience and mistakes, and doesn't have to go through similar awful experiences and lose precious time and energy. A wise person does not waste time and effort easily or lightly. He or she looks first at the most available resources around and makes good use of them. A wise person is the one to make it work. Anybody can be the wise person as long as you are willing to learn and pay attention. The wisdom of wellbeing is the very basic important asset we can acquire for ourselves.

In this chapter, we summarize what we have talked about in the previous chapters and list what we can do to stay healthy, young and energetic

1. Things We Should Do Often Or Hopefully Every Day

- Knock and Massage the stomach meridians, massage the Zu-san-li points.

127

Stomach meridians (figure 3-9), belong to the stomach where the generation of our body's energy starts. Well-maintained stomach meridians are general prerequisites for a healthy stomach, spleen, kidneys and all other organs. By knocking and massaging the stomach meridians on both sides, we can keep them open and freely flowing, so the energy and blood can best be sent out to everywhere in the body.

Zu-san-li points are points on the stomach meridians and the number one wellbeing points. Pressing and massaging these two points for 5 to 10 minutes a day will enhance stomach functionality, strengthen immunity, and increase the energy level (Figure 3-11).

- Knocking the gallbladder meridians

The importance of the gallbladder meridians (figure 3-37) is described in Chapter 3, Section 9. The benefit of knocking these meridians is tremendous.

First, the gallbladder and liver are connected, so when we stimulate the gallbladder, it consequently stimulates the liver to secrete bile which is the substance that dissolves fats and cholesterol in the food we eat. This process greatly improves the body's digestion and absorption.

Second, it gives you a healthier liver because it enhances the liver's ability to clean up the blood and produce the body's immune factors.

Third, knocking these meridians will get rid of coldness and unclog the energy pathway along the sides of the body, and the excessive fat piled up on the sides of the upper legs will decrease.

Last, it is easy to do since these meridians are on the

outer sides of the body, so knocking the portions from the sides of the hips to the outer sides of the knees daily is sufficient and easier. If you can do the entire leg, that would be even better. Try 5 to 10 minutes each side, and if bearable, use more force. Since the most active time of these meridians is 11 pm to1 am, doing this at night before going to bed will be the most effective.

- Foot bath: There are very few acupuncture points on the bottom of the feet, but, almost every part of the body has a reflection area there. Figures 5-2 to 5-6 show these reflections areas. Chinese Medicine doctors can tell which part of your body is not well just by touching your feet. They treat the problems by treating the corresponding areas on the bottom of the feet (see the next section for a discussion of the foot reflection areas).

We don't have to memorize what and where these areas are. The simplest and effective technique is to do a foot bath every day for 30 minutes before going to bed. Use a tall container, so you can immerse more portions of your lower legs. The water temperature depends on your tolerance, but do use the hottest water that you can comfortably tolerate.

As we discussed in Chapter three, there are six meridians starting from or ending at each foot, and all their primary acupuncture points are below the ankles. Foot bathing can active the original energy within the meridians by warming up the primary points and freeing up the energy and blood inside the Jingluos from bottom to top. You'll find yourself sweating after a while. The benefits of a foot bath are tremendous and include a good night's sleep, which all need and enjoy.

- Foot massage: In addition to the foot bath, a foot massage is a great way to stimulate the organ reflection areas on the bottom of the feet. It is very easy. Just rub the bottoms and sides of your feet with your hands for several minutes, it will be nice and warm and help to normalize organ functions. If you want to do a little more, review Figures 5-2 to 5-6 in the next section carefully. Try to find the areas for a specific organ. If anywhere it feels more painful when pressed, press and massage that area for a longer time.

- One foot standing: This sounds easy, right? But wait until you try it. This is what you do. Standing with your hands hanging naturally on the sides, CLOSE your eyes and lift one foot (no need to lift it too high, as long as it is not on the floor). Closing your eyes is the key here, because, when you are able to see, the balance of the body is actually adjusted by the reference objects your eyes see. If you can't see, the body's balance will be controlled by the brain nerves by balancing all the organs. Therefore, you have to concentrate, so the energy and blood can flow down to the standing foot. There are six meridians passing through each leg, so by doing this foot standing, the weaker meridians get worked and strengthened. In the beginning, you probably won't be able to stand for 5 seconds without touching the floor. You should be able to do it longer and longer, however, if you keep trying.

This exercise is very effective for prevent and relieve high blood pressure, diabetes, back pain, neck pain, cerebellum disorders, senile dementia, and sleeplessness. If you always have cold feet, one foot standing will offer fast help.

A one or two minute of one-foot-standing every day will prevent most aging diseases. Again, it is all about normalizing the body's energy and blood flow. When they are free and smooth, there will be no health problems.

- Abdomen Pushing

  Abdomen pushing, as we introduced in the last chapter, is a terrific way to clean up three types of waste in the body: dirty air, dirty water, and old feces. A clean environment does not attract bacteria which causes disease. Like we always clean our houses or other places, our inner bodies also need to be cleaned. Lying on the bed, using both hands, press on the abdomen and slide down, from the chest all way down below the bellybutton. It is best to do it before sleep at night and before you get up in the morning for 5 minutes each time.

  This pushing also massages the conception vessel, stomach meridians, kidney meridians, spleen meridians and liver meridians all at once!

- Massage the pericardium meridians

  Anyone who is over 35 should massage the pericardium meridians (Chapter 3, Section 9, Figure 3-32). It can keep your heart healthy and is a life-saving action. You might not have a heart problem right now, and that's wonderful. If you regularly massage the pericardium meridians, you can stay that way.

Half an hour after dinner or around 7 to 9 o'clock in the evening is a good time to massage the pericardium meridians. They are the center lines of the inner arms, from the middle fingers to the chest. Gently massage and pat them for 3 to 5 minutes on each arm.

- Knee walking

    Legs are usually the first part of the body to show the aging signs as you get older. That's because less and less of the body's energy and blood are able to travel down the legs. Knee walking is an effective way to retrieve energy and send blood to the knee area very quickly. It makes one foot standing a lot easier if you draw energy and blood down to the very bottom of the feet. When legs and the meridians passing through the legs are full of energy and fresh blood, they become strong and all the problems related to energy and blood deficiency are gone using natural means. During the process, built-up fat on the thighs is also flushed away.

    A simple 20 minutes of knee walking daily can cure knee problems, leg problems, and back pain. It also helps you to lose weight and strengthens the liver. Use a mat and walk with your knees on it, is that simple! If your knees hurt, use more cushions and walk slowly or don't walk in the beginning, you'll be used to it later.

- Back pinching

    Back pinching (Figure 3-28) stimulates the bladder meridians (Chapter 3, Section 7) located on the back. Since these meridians are the body's major detoxification channels and have connections to all the major organs though the passage points, it is vital to make them strong and energetic. Doing so will have significant benefits for your overall health condition. As the body's own ability of resisting and curing diseases gets stronger, many unpleasant symptoms will disappear. See 'Section 19: lower back pain' in Chapter 4 and Figure 3-28 for details.

- Abdomen breathing

  This is a fantastic way to boost your energy level and increase your metabolism. Stand and relax with your mind concentrating on the Qi-hai point (Figure 3-43) which is 1.5 Cun below the belly button. Inhale deeply and slowly through the nose to bring the lower abdomen upwards. Stop for a few seconds, and then exhale through the mouth slowly (or quickly) and completely. Repeat several times. If you do 5 to 10 minutes of such exercise, you will have plenty of energy. Do not do abdomen breathing immediately after meals, wait at least one hour.

- Facie and Neck Massage

  There are many meridians going through the face and neck and many acupuncture points in these areas. Memorizing all of them is not practical for most of us, the simplest way to stimulate these points is to gently massage the entire face and neck with both hands to let both energy and blood flow more freely and smoothly, You will have radiant face color and younger skin.

- Comb Hair

  Combing hair is a wonderful way to massage and stimulate the many acupuncture points on the head. The governor vessel, bladder meridians and gallbladder meridians are also massaged. Doing combing will improve the blood circulation on the head, clear the mind, reduce grey hair and prevent hair loss and/or re-grow hair.

- Ear Massage

There are not only a lot of acupuncture points on the ears, but they also reflect the body's health. The ears have reflection areas for almost all the organs and many body parts. Thus, treating disease though ear points is one of the important healing methods in Chinese Medicine. Rubbing and massaging the ears on a regular bases enhances the body's immune ability.

- Hand Rubbing

Like the feet and ears, the hands also reflect the body's health. There are many reflection areas on both of the hands.

Rub both hands to get better energy and blood circulation and increase the body's ability to fight disease.

- Rubbing to warm the lower back

Warm the hands by rubbing them against each other before rubbing the lower back. From Figure 5-1 we can see, at middle of the back, there is the Ming-men point which belongs to the governor vessel (Figure 3-47). On its sides are Shen-shu points, they belong to the bladder meridians (Figure 4-13) and are the kidneys passage points. All these 3 points strengthen the kidneys and support strong vitality and sexuality.

Below them, there are 4 points on each side of the bladder meridians are called Shang-liao point, Ci-liao point, Zhong-liao point and Xia-liao point (meaning upper Liao, second Liao, middle Liao and lower Liao, and Liao means the gap between the bones). These 8 points on both sides together are called 8-Liao points.

For women, they normalize the functionalities of the uterus and ovary. They treat menstruation problems and many female diseases. When the uterus and ovary work well, that means youth for women.

For men, the 8-Liao points treat impotence, involuntary ejaculation. They normalize and strength sexuality.

For both men and women, the 8-Liao points can treat urinary system problems.

Do the rub-to-warm from the Ming-men all the way to the 8-Liao points for 10 to 20 minutes daily.

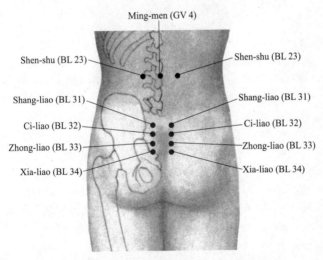

Figure 5-1 (the Ming-men, Shen-shu and 8-Liao points)

2. Feet Reflection Areas

The next 5 figures show the organ reflection areas on the both feet from the bottoms to the backs and to the sides.

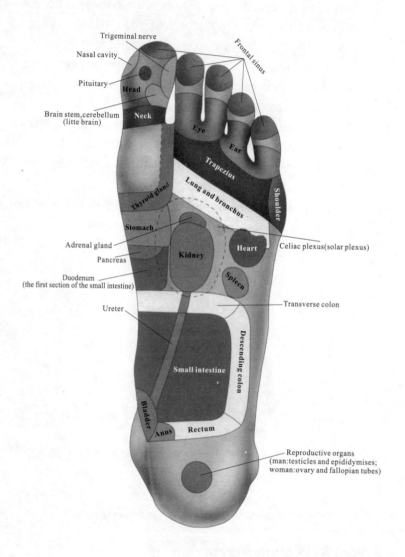

Figure 5-2 (left foot bottom reflection areas)

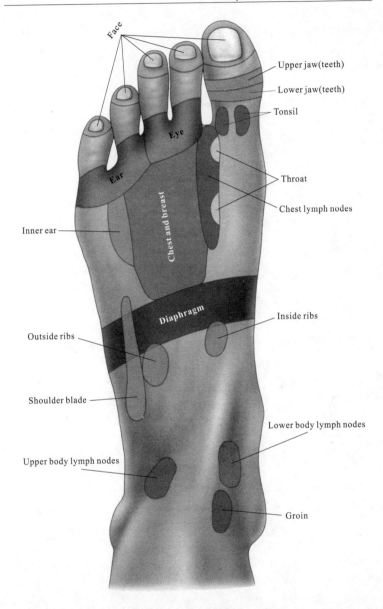

Figure 5-3 (left foot back reflection areas)

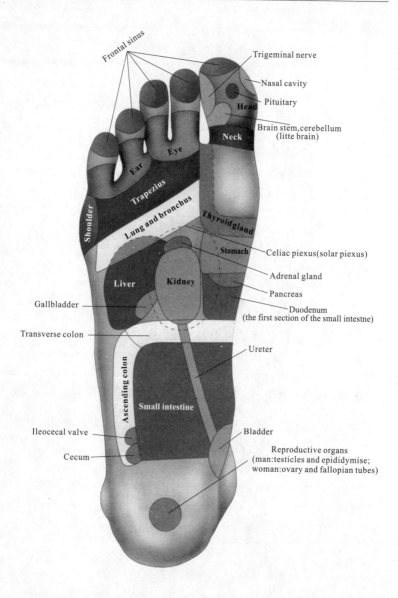

Figure 5-4 (right foot bottom reflection areas)

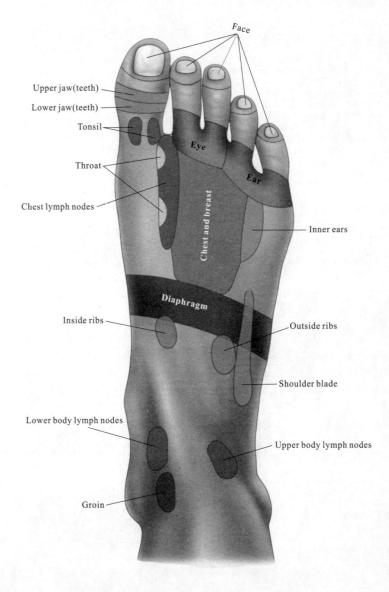

Figure 5-5 (right foot back reflection areas)

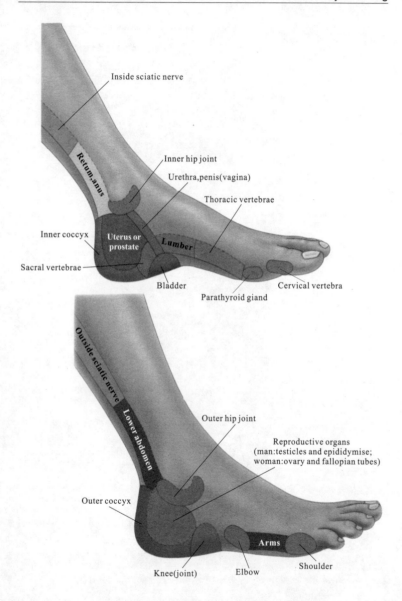

Figure 5-6 (left & right feet sides reflection areas)

3. The Acupuncture Points You Need To Know

There are more then 360 acupuncture points on the human body, it is unpractical for us to memorize all of them of course. We list about 20 points that are the most used and most mentioned. Being familiar with these points is an important step to build wellness using Jingluo therapy.

The easiest and most important way to find and understand acupuncture points is to go with the meridians (Jingluos). In Chapter 3, we listed all the acupuncture points on sketches for each meridian. For your convenience and easier look-up, we put the pictures of all 14 meridians together in the appendix I and all the acupuncture points we used in the appendix II at the end of the book. If you need or want to learn more, go to Chapter 3 or appendix for further reference.

- Zu-san-li

   These are the number one wellbeing points. There are two of them, one on each leg, and they belong to the stomach meridians. A 5-minute massage on each daily will greatly improve the stomach's food processing ability and the strengthen body's immune system. Use a little more pressure on these points (Figure 3-11).

- Yong-quan

   These are the number two wellbeing points. There are two of them, one on the bottom of each foot, and they belong to the kidney meridians. These are anti-aging points. Simulating Yong-quan points can induce energy and blood down to the feet, making the legs and feet stronger. Use more pressure on these points. If you don't feel anything when pressing on them, that means the energy is blocked somewhere above the points, and you need to drive them down by knee walking and one foot standing. Then massage the Yong-quan points again (Figure 3-31).

- Tai-xi

  Tai-xi points are the primary points of the kidney meridians, one on each foot. Sometimes they are called the number one nourishing medicine for the body. They can boost energy in the kidneys and kidney meridians, which support the fundamental functions of human life. They can prevent and cure kidney problems, memory loss, senile dementia, sexuality problems, irregular menstruation, sleeplessness, high blood pressure, asthma, and more. A daily 3-to 5-minute massage on each will be very beneficial (Figure 3-30).

- Bai-hui

  This point belongs to the governor vessel, on the top of the head. It is the highest point on the body, and is a very effective point to clear the mind. It can also lift the body's Yang energy and better energy circulation in the head. It has many capabilities for preventing and curing diseases: headache, stroke, craziness, sleeplessness, memory loss, etc (Figure 3-48).

- He-gu

  This is one of the very important wellbeing points. There are two of them, one on each hand, and they belong to the large intestine meridians. They can be used for headache, sore throat, cold, constipation, etc. They improve immunity and are great pain killers

(Figure 3-6).

- Shou-san-li

These belong to the large intestine meridians, one on each arm, and are important wellbeing points. They lie along the extension line of the index fingers on the thumb side, 2 Cuns below the elbow lines (Figure 5-7). The points deals with arm and shoulder problems, stomach aches and other aches and also strengthen the body's immune ability.

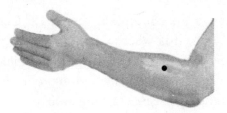

Figure 5-7 (the Shou-san-li point - LI 10)

- Tian-shu

Belong to the stomach meridians, one on each side of the bellybutton. They are the terminals where nutrition and waste are separated and turn to different ways. These are the key points for preventing and curing stomach diseases, constipation, diarrhea (Figure 3-12).

- Tan-zhong

Belongs to the conception vessel, it is the key point for breast health. It can soothe and pacify an upset and depressed heart, when massage this point, do it in a clockwise or downward motion (Figure 3-45).

- Zhong-wan

Belongs to the conception vessel, it normalizes the

function of the stomach and intestines (Figure 4-17).

- Shen-que

  It is in the middle of the bellybutton, belongs to the conception vessel. This is a major wellbeing point, regularly pressing and massaging this point can boost body's original energy, better your health. Moxibustion for 10 to 20 minutes or 100 times press daily are good ways to take care of this point (Figure 3-44). Do not use needles on this point.

- Qi-hai

  Belongs to the conception vessel, 1.5 Cun below the bellybutton. It is where the original energy stays, abdomen breath is a great way to stimulate this point and increases metabolism and improves body's ability of fighting diseases (Figure 3-43).

  Stand and relax, gently press Qi-hai point, inhale deeply and slowly with the nose to bring the lower abdomen up, stop for a few seconds, and then exhale with the mouth slowly (or quickly) and completely, repeat for several times. Do not do it immediately after meals.

- Guan-yuan

  This is the number one wellbeing point for strong sexuality, it is also the key point for general wellbeing and longevity. Moxibustion for 10 to 20 minutes daily in winter is the best way to take care of it, pressing and massaging is also effective (Figure 3-42).

- Tai-chong

  These are the primary points of the liver meridians. They are the most crucial detoxifying processors in the body. They can ease the liver, normalize the energy flow in the liver and liver meridians. If you are easy to get angry, massaging these points will calm you down. They are used at so many occasions and treat many types of diseases (Figure 3-40).

- Nei-guan

  They belong to the pericardium meridians. Their responsibilities involve heart, stomach and lungs. High blood pressure, coronary heart disease, irregular heart beat, trouble sleeping, depression, stomachache, etc. are all within their reach (Figure 3-34).

- San-yin-jiao

  Belong to the spleen meridians, one on each leg. They are where the three Yin meridians meet: liver meridians, kidney meridians and spleen meridians, therefore they can be used for preventing and treating many diseases related to all these meridians. They are the key points for curing many woman diseases. They are also effective for relieving stomach bloating, sexuality problems, sleeplessness, knee problems and etc (Figure 3-17).

- Shen-shu

  These are the kidney passage points on the bladder meridians. They are very effective for strengthening the kidneys. Use both hands to rub the areas around these two points to transmit the warmness to the kidneys, 200 times each session is adequate (Figure 4-13).

- Ming-men

  It is on the governor vessel, centerline of the back and on the same level with the bellybutton. It is also an important kidney nourishing point, helps to prevent and cure lower back problems, libido problems for men and menstruation problems for women (Figure 3-47).

- Tian-zong

  They belong to the small intestine meridians and are really useful for treating shoulder and cervical neck pains, those who work long hours in front of computers should especially remember these two points (Figure 3-25).

- Ji-quan

  Two points and one under each armpit, they belong to the heart meridians, are responsible for normalizing heart beat rate, easing nervousness, curing difficulty raising arms and relieving depression (Figure 3-21).

- Feng-chi

  They are on the neck and belong to the gallbladder meridians. They are very helpful for treating cold, headache, migraine and other cold air related symptoms (Figure 4-2).

- Tai-yuan

  These are the primary points of the lung meridians, one on each hand. These points can solve short of breath very well, they also deal with cough, sore throat, irregular heart beat, weak pulse, chest pain etc (Figure 3-2).

- Gong-sun

  They belong to the spleen meridians, on the sides of the feet. Very useful for treating the chest and abdomen problems as well as female problems, such as bloating, abdomen pain, heart pain, stomachache, chest pain, painful menstruation, irregular menstruation, infertility etc. (Figure 3-16).

- Wei-zhong

  They belong to the bladder meridians. Stimulating these points can activate the bladder meridians, unblock the energy and blood flow on the back, therefore cure back pains (Figure 4-29).

- Hou-xi

  They belong to the small intestine meridians (Figure 4-33). Stimulating these points will prevent and relieve neck and back pains effectively, mostly caused by long hour working in front of desks and computers. Just roll your hands on the desk with these points underneath for a few minutes every once a while, it will be very beneficial.

4. About Food

I believe that most people agree that eating habits seriously affect our quality of life, whether you act on the issue or not. We are surrounded by so much tasty, convenient, and yet unhealthy food that without some conscious effort, it is hard to avoid the harmful temptations.

Food is our body's energy source. After it enters the stomach, it is processed and turned into energy that supports our life activities. If the food source is low quality or not suitable for your body, how can you get good energy from it?

There are so many books and publications out there today that try to tell you what foods are nutritious and what ones are not. But not too many people talk about the nature of the foods and how well they fit different individuals.

Even good and nutritious food is not necessarily always good for you if you don't understand your body type or the nature of the food. Different people have different body types. Some people belong to the hot type, some belong to the cold type, some are in between. Foods also have different characters, generally speaking, plants grown in a cold environment are mostly a hotter nature, and those grow in a hot environment are mostly a colder nature. These are the modes for survival and the brilliant way that all things are created.

For example, water melons and bananas are tropical plants or only grow in summer, they are cold in nature. If a person with a cold type body eats too many (even in the summer time), these foods bring down the inside body temperature even more. Coldness slows down energy and blood flow. By now, you should know how much unpleasantness that can cause for you.

Today, technology and transportation made it possible for people live anywhere eat food grown anywhere else and at any time. That does not necessary mean it is all great for us. Nature has different climate zones and different seasons. Different creations are made to fit the particular areas or particular seasons. This has been the law of nature for millions and millions of years. A human being is part of nature, so only by following nature's rules and living harmoniously with nature can you survive in peace.

This idea sounds very primitive, right? The truth is, the evolution of human body has been much much slower then the development of science and technology. It is calculated by hundreds of thousands even millions of years. I am sure that several hundred thousand years later, our bodies are so developed to take whatever we eat now and process it well. However, that's under the assumption that human beings still exist and they stay on the same diet as today. Until that day comes, our bodies will still be the same as our ancestors several thousands years ago. If we want to live well, the best thing is to meet these needs, survive, and thrive peacefully with them.

- How do we know what our body types are?

  In Chinese Medicine, the type of body can be complicated, but there are some general guidelines we can use here to make sense of our own bodies. If you have more 'yes' then 'no' answers to the following 11 statement, your body is a hotter type. Otherwise you have a colder type of body:

  (1) You always like to drink cold drinks even in winter.

  (2) The tongue is a dark red color.

  (3) Talk fast and clearly.

  (4) Have plenty of saliva.

  (5) Always have warm hands.

  (6) Cheeks are reddish.

  (7) Often open eyes widely unintentionally.

  (8) Normal body temperature is above 97.3 degree Fahrenheit.

  (9) It's not easy to sit still, like to shift body left and right.

  (10) Smaller body frame and appears to have less weight then actual weight.

  (11) Muscles on the lower legs are looser, easy to pinch.

- How do we know the real nature of foods?

  There are many references and books give this information, you have to check for each particular food you are interested in for its nature.

We list below some foods with their characters as an example:

1) Normal natured foods:

Rice, corn, sweet potato, sesame, soy bean, red small bean, black bean; pork, milk, yogurt, scallop, salmon, trout, sea cucumber; plum, pine apple, sunflower seed, peanut, hazel nut, chestnut; wild yam, carrot, potato, mushroom; soy milk, peanut oil, soy bean oil,.

2) Warm natured foods:

Black Rice, sticky rice, broomcorn; beef, lamb, chicken, shrimp; peach, apricot, date, lemon, walnut, papaya, pine tree seed, cherries; green onion, onion, garlic, pumpkin; ginger, brown sugar, coffee.

3) Hot natured foods:

Hot pepper, black pepper.

4) Cool natured foods:

Millet, wheat, mung bean; frog meat; apples, pears, oranges, strawberries, mangos; tomatoes, celery, eggplant, spinach, tofu; green tea, honey, ginseng.

5) Cold natured foods:

Duck, horse meat, crab, octopus, oyster; persimmon, grapefruit, banana, watermelon, kiwifruit; soy sauce.

A hot body type person should not eat too much hot-natured food. If you do, combine with some cold-natured food to bring down the hotness. A cold type body person, should not eat too much cold-natured food; combine with some hot-natured food if you do.

Normal natured foods can be eaten all the time. Eat less warm natured food during summer. Cool natured food can be eaten often in the summer and combined with some warm natured foods in other seasons. Eat as little as possible of cold natured foods, but when you do, add some hot natured food like hot pepper or ginger.

A person's body type can change because of change in life style, the aging process, sickness, or other expected or unexpected factors. No matter what, always keep in mind that a warmer body moves energy and blood better, and a warmer body runs the metabolism more efficiently. Generally, a warmer body means a healthier body.

5. About Sleep

Again, we are living in a body type as old as it was thousands years ago, as old as when our daily activities were oriented by the sun movements, getting up when the sun rises, going to sleep after sundown. Our body is built to consume and regenerate energy and blood based on this kind of use. The best time for our body to regenerate energy, blood, human growth hormone, and other vital elements is after 11 o'clock at night during deep sleep. If you always stay up late, overuse your body and do not give it enough time to rest, your body will not generate the energy and blood for you to stay healthy. After a while, like a machine that is overused, the body will malfunction. If no maintenance is given, it will give up eventually and stop running.

Thus, it only makes sense to have the habit of going to bed early (around 10 pm) and get up early. In that way, you can fully recharge the body every day, and stay energetic all day long.

6. About Coldness

In Chinese medicine, there are six types of evil that cause all illnesses. They are: wind, coldness, dampness, dryness, hotness, and summer heat. Wind moves cold air, therefore, the number one and number two evils are both related to coldness.

In winters, coldness freezes rivers. It will slow down or freeze energy and the blood circulation in our body in the same way. Therefore, it is never a good idea to eat or drink frozen cold food or beverages all the time even if doing so is a pleasant at the moment. It is never a good idea for any-one to dress too sparsely in real cold weather, even if doing so gives you a good look you like.

It is all about energy. Energy is the power that moves our lives. We cannot afford not to pay attention to it! We must respect and honor where our energy comes from in our lives.

Appendix I
The Fourteen Meridians

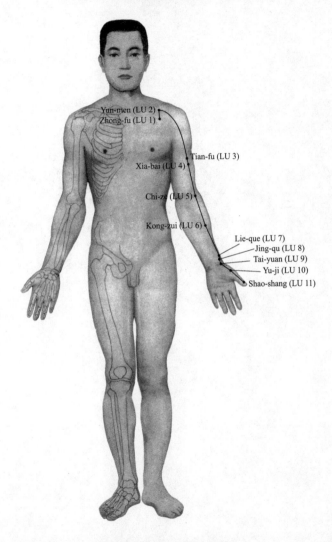

Yun-men (LU 2)
Zhong-fu (LU 1)
Tian-fu (LU 3)
Xia-bai (LU 4)
Chi-ze (LU 5)
Kong-zui (LU 6)
Lie-que (LU 7)
Jing-qu (LU 8)
Tai-yuan (LU 9)
Yu-ji (LU 10)
Shao-shang (LU 11)

Figure 1: the lung meridian
The most active time: 3 am to 5 am
The primary point: Tai-yuan (LU 9)

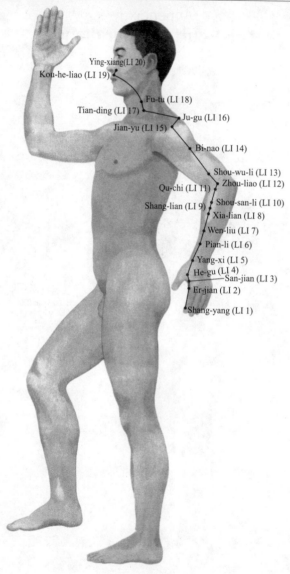

Figure 2: the large intestine meridian
The most active time: 5 am to 7 am
The primary point: He-gu (LI 4)

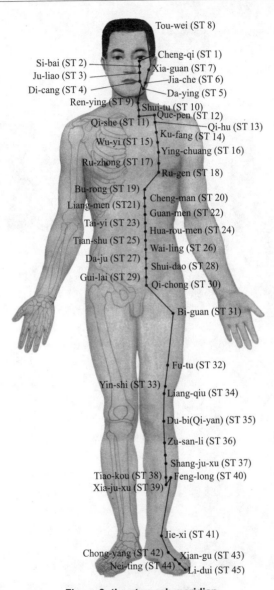

Tou-wei (ST 8)
Cheng-qi (ST 1)
Si-bai (ST 2)
Xia-guan (ST 7)
Ju-liao (ST 3)
Jia-che (ST 6)
Di-cang (ST 4)
Da-ying (ST 5)
Ren-ying (ST 9)
Shui-tu (ST 10)
Que-pen (ST 12)
Qi-she (ST 11)
Qi-hu (ST 13)
Ku-fang (ST 14)
Wu-yi (ST 15)
Ying-chuang (ST 16)
Ru-zhong (ST 17)
Ru-gen (ST 18)
Bu-rong (ST 19)
Cheng-man (ST 20)
Liang-men (ST21)
Guan-men (ST 22)
Tai-yi (ST 23)
Hua-rou-men (ST 24)
Tian-shu (ST 25)
Wai-ling (ST 26)
Da-ju (ST 27)
Shui-dao (ST 28)
Gui-lai (ST 29)
Qi-chong (ST 30)
Bi-guan (ST 31)
Fu-tu (ST 32)
Yin-shi (ST 33)
Liang-qiu (ST 34)
Du-bi(Qi-yan) (ST 35)
Zu-san-li (ST 36)
Shang-ju-xu (ST 37)
Tiao-kou (ST 38)
Feng-long (ST 40)
Xia-ju-xu (ST 39)
Jie-xi (ST 41)
Chong-yang (ST 42)
Xian-gu (ST 43)
Nei-ting (ST 44)
Li-dui (ST 45)

Figure 3: the stomach meridian
The most active time: 7 am to 9 am
The primary point: Chong-yang (ST 42)

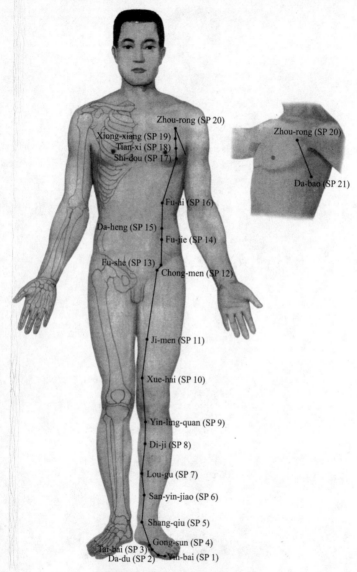

Figure 4: the spleen meridian
The most active time: 9 am to 11 am
The primary point: Tai-bai (SP 3)

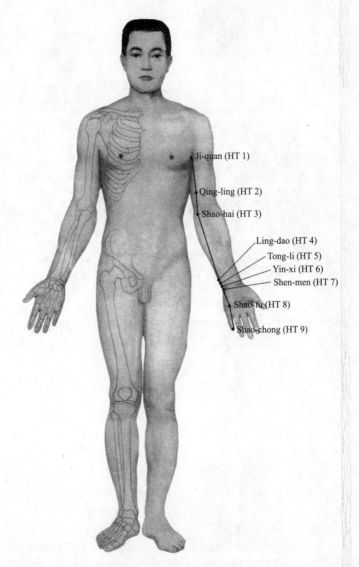

Ji-quan (HT 1)

Qing-ling (HT 2)

Shao-hai (HT 3)

Ling-dao (HT 4)
Tong-li (HT 5)
Yin-xi (HT 6)
Shen-men (HT 7)

Shao-fu (HT 8)

Shao-chong (HT 9)

Figure 5: the heart meridian
The most active time: 11 am to 1 pm
The primary point: Shen-men (HT 7)

157

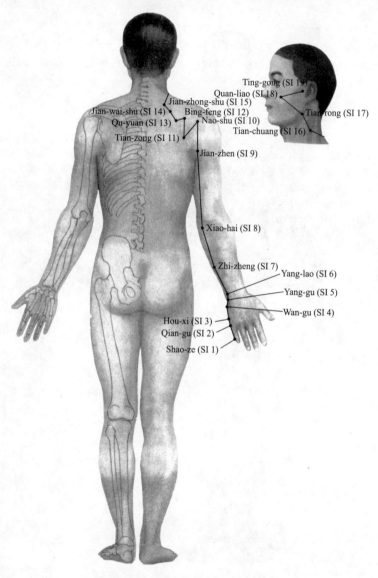

Figure 6: the small Intestine meridian
The most active time: 1 pm to 3 pm
The primary point: Wan-gu (SI 4)

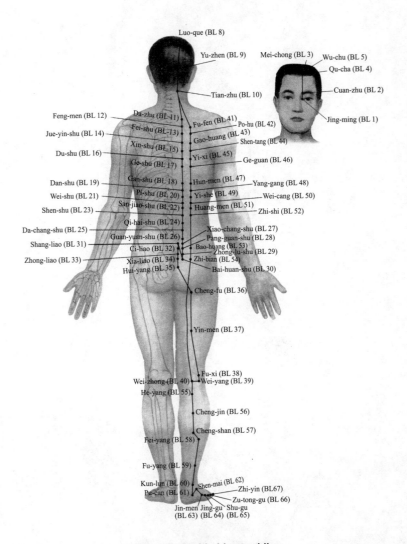

Figure 7: the bladder meridian
The most active time: 3 pm to 5 pm
The primary point: Jing-gu (BL 64)

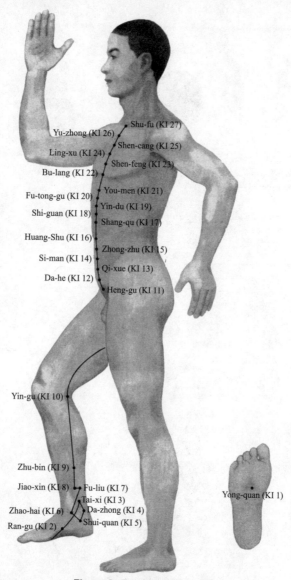

Figure 8: the kidney meridian
The most active time: 5 pm to 7 pm
The primary point: Tai-xi (KI 3)

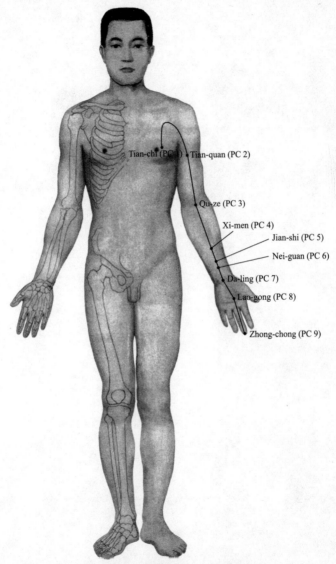

Tian-chi (PC 1)   •Tian-quan (PC 2)

Qu-ze (PC 3)

Xi-men (PC 4)

Jian-shi (PC 5)

Nei-guan (PC 6)

Da-ling (PC 7)

Lao-gong (PC 8)

Zhong-chong (PC 9)

Figure 9: the pericardium meridian
The most active time: 7 pm to 9 pm
The primary point: Da-ling (PC 7)

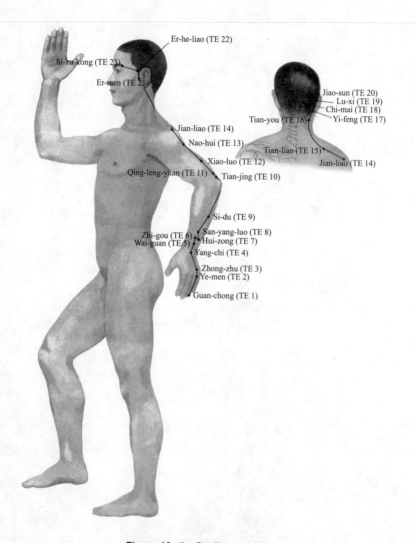

Figure 10: the Sanjiao meridian
The most active time: 9 pm to 11 pm
The primary point: Yang-chi (TE 4)

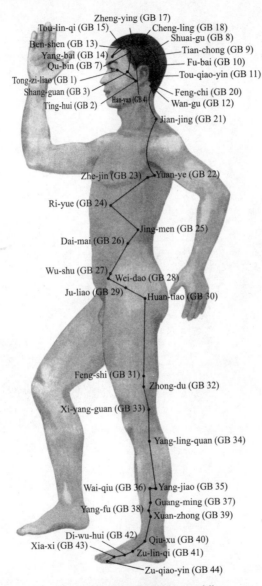

Figure 11: the gallbladder meridian
The most active time: 11 pm to 1 am
The primary point: Qiu-xu (GB 40)

163

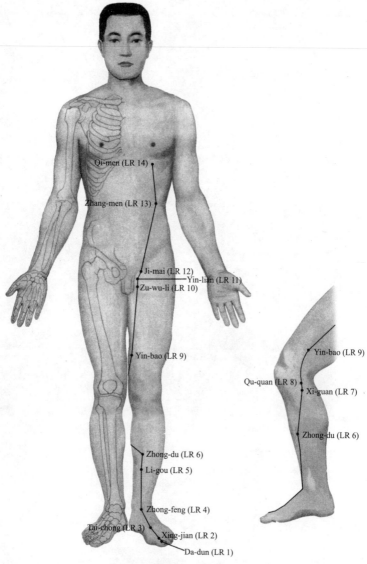

Figure 12: the liver meridian
The most active time: 1 am to 3 am
The primary point: Tai-chong (LR 3)

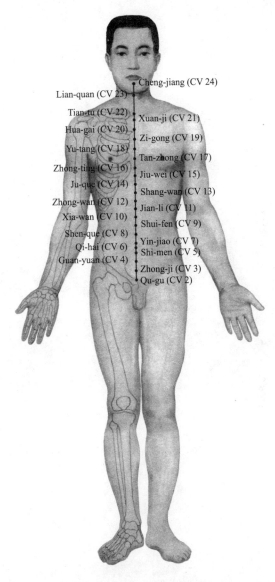

Cheng-jiang (CV 24)
Lian-quan (CV 23)
Tian-tu (CV 22)
Xuan-ji (CV 21)
Hua-gai (CV 20)
Zi-gong (CV 19)
Yu-tang (CV 18)
Tan-zhong (CV 17)
Zhong-ting (CV 16)
Jiu-wei (CV 15)
Ju-que (CV 14)
Shang-wan (CV 13)
Zhong-wan (CV 12)
Jian-li (CV 11)
Xia-wan (CV 10)
Shui-fen (CV 9)
Shen-que (CV 8)
Yin-jiao (CV 7)
Qi-hai (CV 6)
Shi-men (CV 5)
Guan-yuan (CV 4)
Zhong-ji (CV 3)
Qu-gu (CV 2)

Figure 13: the conception vessel

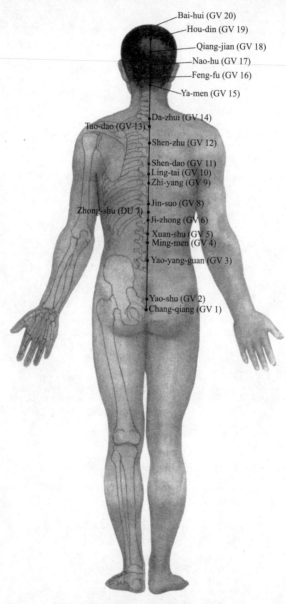

Figure 14: the governor vessel

Appendix II
The Acupuncture Points Used in This Book

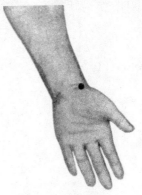

Figure 3-2
(the Tai-yuan point - LU 9)

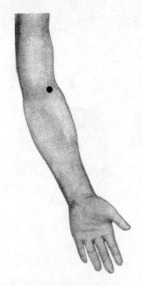

Figure 3-3
(the Chi-ze point - LU 5)

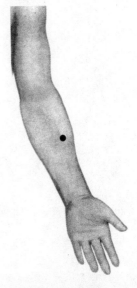

Figure 3-4
(the Kong-zui point - LU 6)

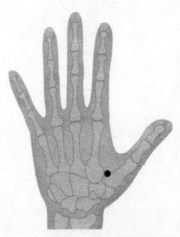

Figure 3-6 (the He-gu point - LI 4)

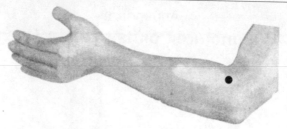

Figure 3-7 (the Qu-chi point - LI 11)

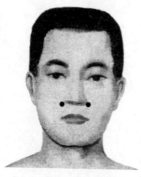

Figure 3-8 (the Ying-xiang points - LI 20)

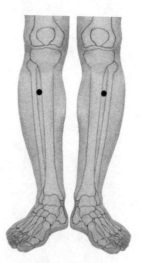

Figure 3-11
(the Zu-san-li points - ST 36)

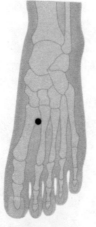

Figure 3-10
(the Chong-yang point - ST 42)

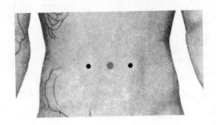

Figure 3-12
(the Tian-shu points - ST 25)

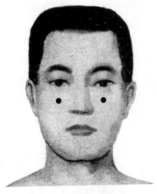

Figure 3-13
(the Si-bai points - ST 2)

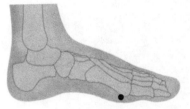

Figure 3-15 (the Tai-bai point - SP 3)

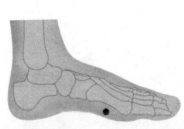

Figure 3-16 (the Gong-sun point - SP 4)

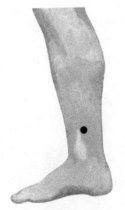

Figure 3-17
(the San-yin-jiao point - SP 6)

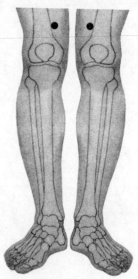

Figure 3-18
(the Xue-hai points - SP 10)

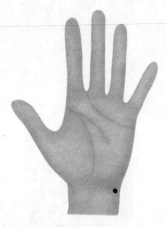

Figure 3-20
(The Shen-men point - HT 7)

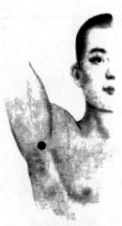

Figure 3-21
(the Ji-quan points - HT 1)

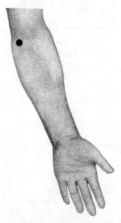

Figure 3-22
(the Shao-hai point - HT 3)

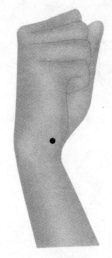

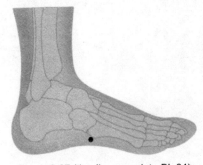

Figure 3-27 (the Jing-gu point - BL 64)

Figure 3-24
(the Wan-gu point - SI 4)

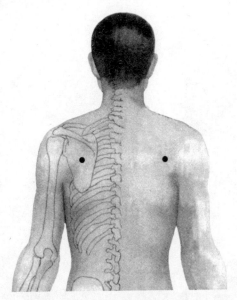

Figure 3-25 (the Tian-zong points - SI 11)

171

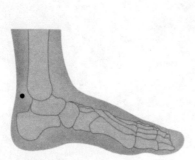

Figure 3-30 (the Tai-xi point - KI 3)

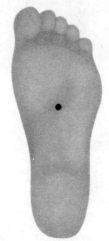

Figure 3-31
(the Yong-quan point - KI 1)

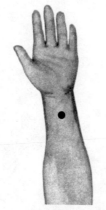

Figure 3-34
(the Nei-guan point - PC 6)

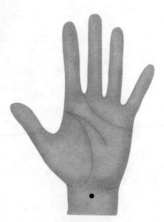

Figure 3-33
(the Da-ling point - PC 7)

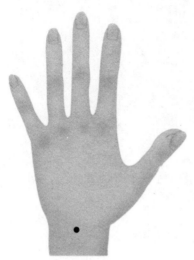

Figure 3-36 (the Yang-chi point - TE 4)

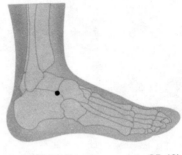

Figure 3-38 (the Qiu-xu point - GB 40)

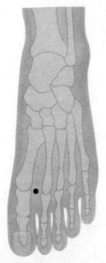

Figure 3-40
(the Tai-chong point - LR 3)

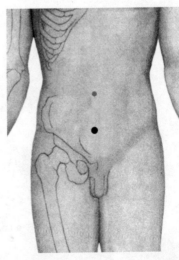

Figure 3-42 (the Guan-yuan point - CV 4)

173

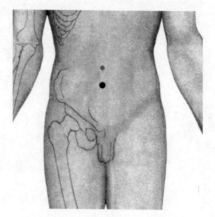

Figure 3-43 (the Qi-hai point - CV 6)

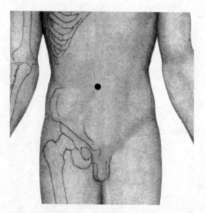

Figure 3-44 (the Shen-que point - CV 8)

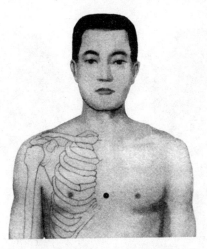

Figure 3-45 (the Tan-zhong point - CV 17)

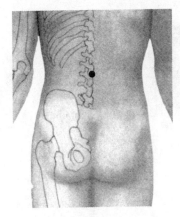

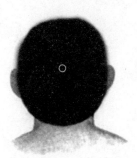

Figure 3-47
(the Ming-men point - GV 4)

Figure 3-48
(the Bai-hui point - GV 20)

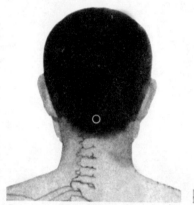 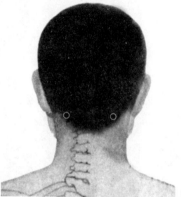

Figure 4-1
(the Feng-fu point - GV 16)

Figure 4-2
(the Feng-chi points - GB 20)

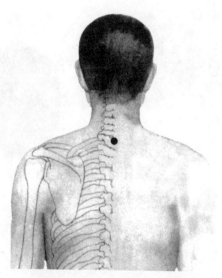

Figure 4-3 (the Da-zhui point - GV 14)

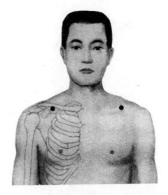

Figure 4-4
(the Yun-men point - LU 2)

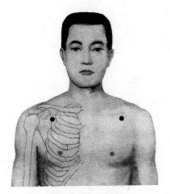

Figure 4-5
(the Zhong-fu point - LU 1)

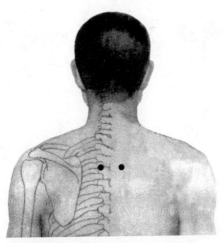

Figure 4-6 (the Fei-shu point - BL 13)

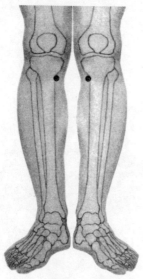

Figure 4-7
(the Yin-ling-quan points - SP 9)

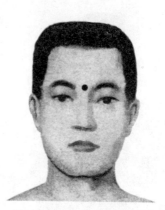

Figure 4-8 (the Yin-tang point)

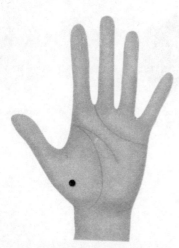

Figure 4-9 (the Yu-ji point - LU 10)

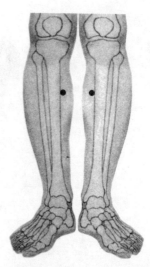

Figure 4-10 (the Di-ji points - SP 8)

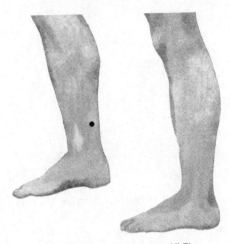

Figure 4-11 (the Fu-liu point - KI 7)

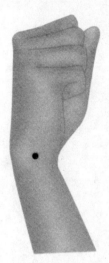

Figure 4-12
(the Yang-gu point - SI 5)

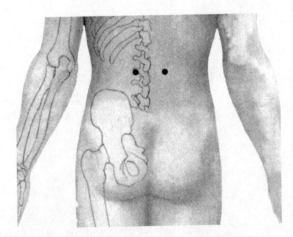

Figure 4-13 (the Shen-shu points - BL 23)

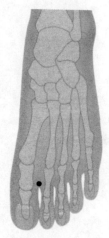

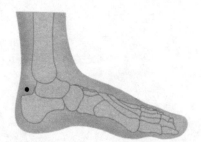

Figure 4-15 (the Shui-quan point - KI 5)

Figure 4-14
(the Xing-jian point - LR 2)

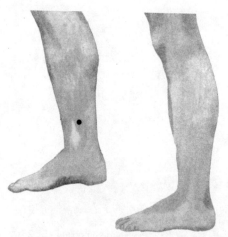

Figure 4-16 (the Jiao-xin point - KI 8)

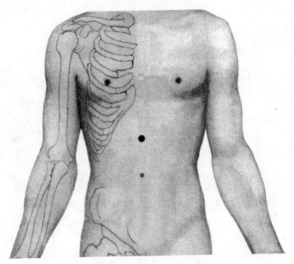

Figure 4-17 (the Zhong-wan point - CV12)

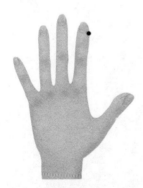

Figure 4-18
(the Shang-yang point - LI 1)

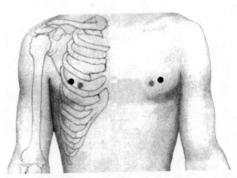

Figure 4-19 (the Tian-chi points - PC 1)

181

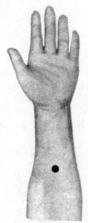

Figure 4-20
(the Xi-men point - PC 4)

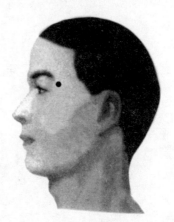

Figure 4-22
(the Tai-yang point - EX-HN 5)

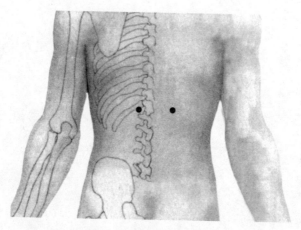

Figure 4-21 (the Pi-shu point - BL 20)

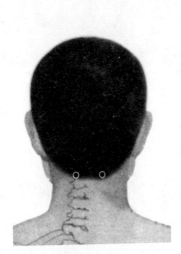

Figure 4-23
(the Tian-zhu points - BL 10)

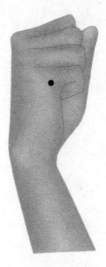

Figure 4-24
(the Qian-gu point - SI 2)

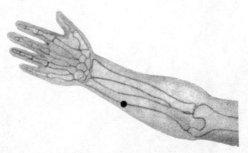

Figure 4-25 (the Zhi-zheng point - SI 7)

183

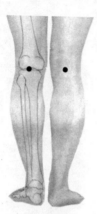

Figure 4-29
(the Wei-zhong points-BL 40)

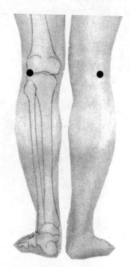

Figure 4-30
(the Wei-yang points - BL 39)

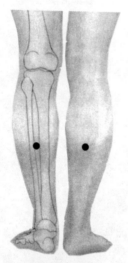

Figure 4-31
(the cheng-shan points - BL 57)

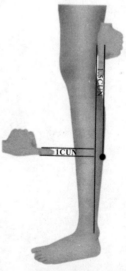

Figure 4-32
(the Fei-yang point - BL 58)

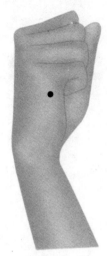

Figure 4-33
(the Hou-xi point - SI 3)

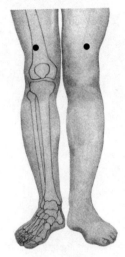

Figure 4-34
(the Liang-qiu points - ST 34)

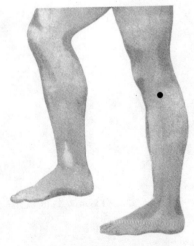

Figure 4-35
(the Yang-ling-quan point-GB 34)

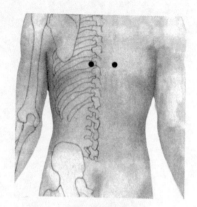

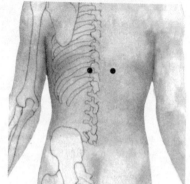

Figure 4-36
(the Ge-shu points - BL 17)

Figure 4-37
(the Gan-shu points - BL 18)

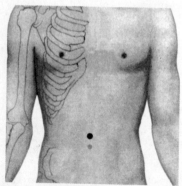

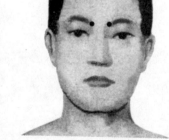

Figure 4-38 (the Shui-fen point - CV 9) Figure 4-39 (the Cuan-zhu points - BL 2)

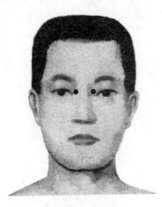

Figure 4-40
(the Jing-ming points - BL 1)

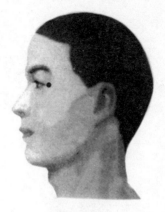

Figure 4-41
(the Tong-zi-liao point - GB 1)

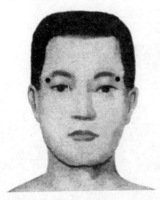

Figure 4-42
(the Si-zhu-kong points - TE 23)

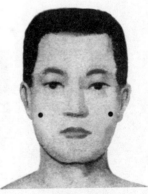

Figure 4-43
(the Quan-liao points - SI 18)

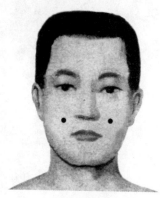

Figure 4-44
(the Ju-liao points - ST 3)

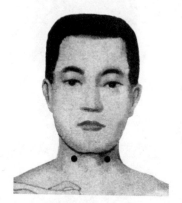

Figure 4-45
(the Ren-ying points - ST 9)

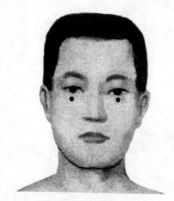

Figure 4-46 (the Cheng-qi points - St 1)

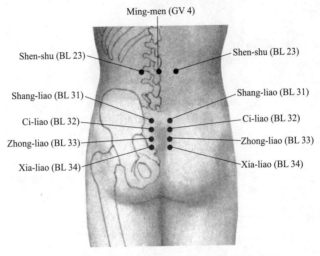

Figure 5-1 (the Ming-men, Shen-shu and 8-Liao points)

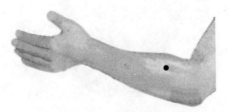

Figure 5-7 (the Shou-san-li point - LI 10)

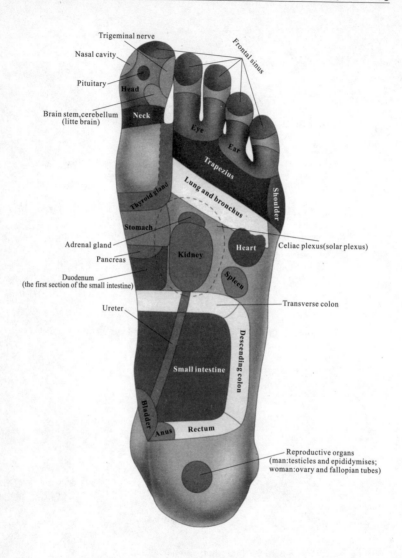

Figure 5-2 (left foot bottom reflection areas)

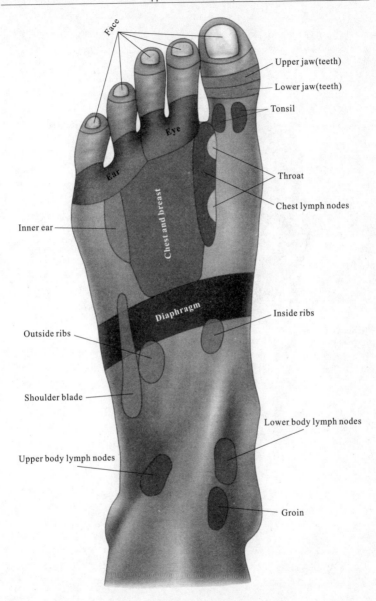

Figure 5-3 (left foot back reflection areas)

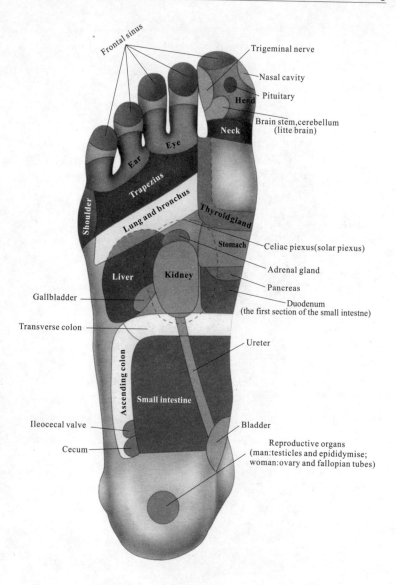

Figure 5-4 (right foot bottom reflection areas)

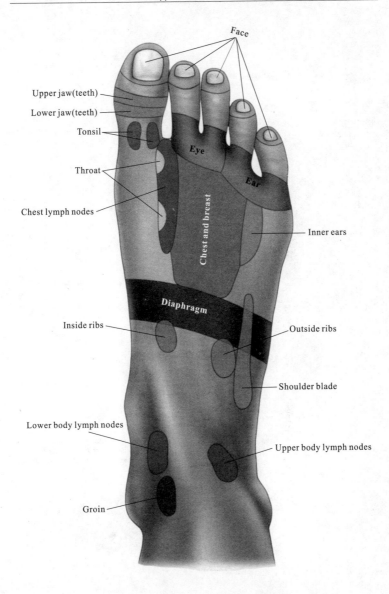

Figure 5-5 (right foot back reflection areas)

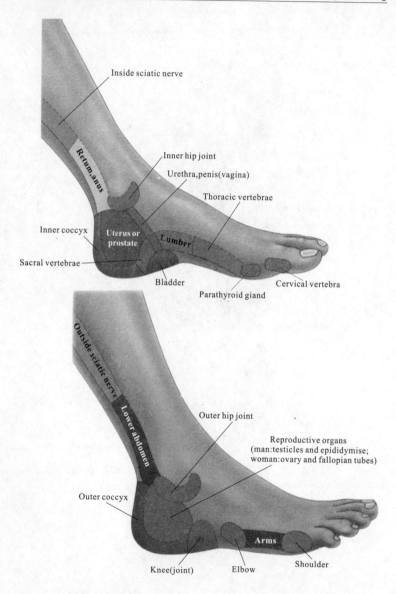

Figure 5-6 (left & right feet sides reflection areas)

References

1. "The handbook of how to use Jingluos in human body" by Xiao Yansheng. Publisher: the oriental press

2. "The handbook of special effect acupuncture points" by Xiao Yansheng. Publisher: the phoenix publishing and media network, Jiangsu literature and art publishing company

3. "The Whole body message illustration" by Chinese medicine health care group. Publisher: China light industry press

4. "You can help yourself better then the doctors can" by Zhong li ba ren. Publisher: China press of traditional Chinese medicine

5. "You can help yourself better then the doctors can (2)" by Zhong li ba ren. Publisher: the phoenix publishing and media network, Jiangsu literature and art publishing company

6. "You can help yourself better then the doctors can (3)" by Zhong li ba ren. Publisher: the phoenix publishing and media network, Jiangsul iterature and art press

7. "The great medicines in human body " by Wu Guozhong. Publisher: the phoenix publishing and media network, Jiangsu literature and art press

8. "The wisdom of not being sick" by Ma yueling, Publisher: the phoenix publishing and media network, Jiangsu literature and art press

9. "The user's manual for human body" by Wu qing-

zhong. Publisher: Guangdong province publishing group, the flower city press

10. "Live until the natural year" by Wu Guozhong. Publisher: Jilin science and technology press

11. "The hands and feet massage illustration" by Chinese medicine health care group. Publisher: China light industry press

12. The Latest international standard wall chart of acupuncture points

13. "The Yellow Emperor's Classics of Internal Medicine"

14. www.wikipedia.org

15. "The discipline of not being sick" by Zhang Heyao. Publisher: the phoenix publishing and media network, Jiangsu literature and art press

Index

INDEX

Abnormal skin blood
  circulation, 21
Acupuncture, 11
Acupuncture point, 2,11,12,13,
  141
Acute bronchitis, 47
Agitation, 29
Angina, 37,53,102
Arm and shoulder pain, 21
Arthritis, 47,71
Asthma, 20,21,47,78,80,81,82,
  142
Back pain, 35,47,51,64,71,114,
  131,147
Back pinching, 47,48,113,116,
  132
Bad temper, 64
Bai-hui, 73,103,111,142
Beauty Matters, 118
Belt Vessel, 7,95,98
Bianque, 9
Bitterness in the mouth, 61
Bladder, 5,45
Bladder meridian, 5,6,45,75,90,
  96,113,114
Bloating, 29,33,35,89,93,107,
  146
Body types, 148,149
Breast diseases, 70

Breast problems, 61,87
Bronchitis, 21,25,47,78
Cervical neck pains, 47,146
Chest congestion, 64,66,70
Chest pain, 21,22,53,80,146
Chi-ze, 21,22,80
Cholecystitis, 47
Chong Vessel, 7,71
Chong-yang, 29
Chronic tracheitis, 21
Cold, 21,25,47,58,76
Coldness, 15,16,96,99,128,148,
  152
Conception Vessel, 7,8,12,66,
  81,87,131
Constipation, 25,31,33,43,58,96,
  97,105,142
Coronary heart disease, 37,102,
  145
Cough, 20,21,25,70,78,80,146
Craziness, 29,142
Cun, 13,14,17,19
Cupping, 16,80,96,107
Da-ling, 53,55,103
Depression, 37,39,55,64,99,100,
  145,146
Diabetes, 58,83,131
Diarrhea, 31,33,105,143
Digestive system, 23,32,47,59,

197